I0492879

Easy-to-Hard Sudoku Vol. 1

250 Puzzles of Mixed Difficulty Levels

RAINA CLAYTON

Copyright © Bizcom AP, 2016

Disclaimer

All Rights Reserved. No part of this book may be reproduced or transmitted in any form or by any means, mechanical or electronic, including photocopying or recording, or by any information storage and retrieval system, or transmitted by email without permission in writing from the publisher. This book is for entertainment purposes only. The views expressed are those of the author alone.

Table of Contents

Introduction

This book is the first volume of a series on Easy-to-Hard Sudoku. It comes in a relatively large dimensions of 8" x 10" and with only four puzzles on each page. The primary purpose of this is to provide decent size puzzles with sufficient blank spaces for writing notes and for ease of use. If you are looking for books with slightly smaller dimension, there is a portable travel edition that form part of this series. Details of this can be found at the end of the book. Do note that all puzzles are unique in all volumes and editions. You will not find the exact same puzzle repeated in any volume or edition of this series.

Another feature is that the puzzles are grouped in a range of difficulties from the beginner's level to the more advanced level. There is also a section consisting of puzzles with random difficulties resulting in five levels; namely (1) easy, (2) medium, (3) hard, (4) very hard, and (5) random. This is to cater to a larger range of users' interests and experiences. We have included additional puzzles to compensate for users who might decide that a certain difficulty level is either too easy or too difficult and will therefore not be making full use of the entire book. A total of 250 puzzles are provided in each volume of 'Easy-to-Hard Sudoku'.

Do note also that all puzzles within each Difficulty Level are assigned a difficulty factor ranging between 0.01 and 1.00 (the higher the value, the more difficult the puzzle). This additional information might be of interests to some readers but if this does not apply to you, just ignore them.

Solutions to all the puzzles are provided towards the later part of the book.

Beginners Guide

What is Sudoku?

Sudoku is a logic-based puzzle of number-placement. It is not a guessing game so a true Sudoku puzzle will have only one completely correct solution. There can be no ambiguity as each number (or digit) has a single right location it must reside in. If not for this requirement, a player will be forced to guess which location on the grid to choose thus changing the puzzle into a game of chance.

Sudoku puzzles are really easy to understand and can be very addictive. All that is required is to simply fill the empty grid with numbers according to the few simple rules of the game. Solving these puzzles can be extremely engaging and fun to populate the grids. Some can be completed relatively fast while others might take much more time to solve. There is no need for any knowledge of mathematics; just an inquisitive mind and a pencil. The numbers used are purely symbolic with no quantitative value.

The beauty of these puzzles is that they can be played by people of all ages and abilities.

Each standard Sudoku puzzle is a 9x9 grid divided into nine smaller 3x3 blocks. Each puzzle begins with some pre-filled cells. The objective is to completely fill the 9x9 grid with numbers (ranging from 1 to 9) such that each row, each column, and each of the 3×3 grids that together form the larger 9×9 grid, contains all of the numbers from 1 to 9. The player uses the pre-filled numbers to help in finding the correct numbers for the empty grids.

It is necessary to highlight that no number from 1 to 9 can be repeated in any column or row. However, it is perfectly fine for numbers to appear more than once along the diagonals.

An additional information of interest: Sudoku is a Japanese word meaning 'single number'.

The Rules of Sudoku

The rules are very clear and straight forward:

- You are to fill in to every cell in the grid, a number 1 to 9.
- Each number can only be used once in each row, each column, and in each of the 3x3 boxes.

To successfully solve Sudoku puzzles, you need to be focused, patient, and disciplined. Do not try guessing as it will not work. For the beginners, with a bit of experience and practicing on the easier puzzles, you will very quickly get to make rapid progress. You will naturally advance to higher difficulty Sudoku without even realizing it.

How to Solve Sudoku Puzzles

This segment is meant to provide some tips for the beginners.
You can begin solving a Sudoku puzzle from anywhere within the 9x9 grid. Over time you would know your preferred style of play and this will come quite fast.

Some questions you might ask yourself as you approach solving the puzzles:
- Where could I place the number X (any number from 1 to 9) in this column / this row / this box?
  (Visually scan the existing numbers already in the column / row / box and see if you can detect a potential number for any of the empty cell.)
- What number could I place in this cell?
  (If you can determine a correct number, put it in.)
- Which column / row / box is getting full, and can I fill the remaining cells now?

A few additional tips:
- The puzzle might appear difficult in the beginning. But as you begin to fill a few cells, it quickly gets easier as you continue making progress.
- The correct solution is there somewhere. Don't give up yet.
- From beginner to very advanced levels, there is no need to make guesses. It's all about logical reasoning.

EASY

SUDOKU

Puzzle 1 (Easy, difficulty rating 0.44)

5		2						
4	7			8	2	5	1	
				3	5			
9		5			3			
3	1						5	6
			4			8		9
			5	2				
	2	9	6	1			8	5
						6		7

Puzzle 2 (Easy, difficulty rating 0.35)

				1	2	8	4	5
	1		7				3	
	8		6		9			
2					7	4		
		5				9		
		8	9					2
			1		3		9	
	3				4		8	
1	5	9	2	6				

Puzzle 3 (Easy, difficulty rating 0.44)

9			2					
2						7	5	9
4		8	7					1
	9	4		3				
	8		4	2	5		9	
			6			1	7	
7					8	3		5
8	3	2						7
					2			6

Puzzle 4 (Easy, difficulty rating 0.38)

	9				2	4		
6				9	5	1		
	5			1			3	2
	8	2		6				
7				3				8
				4		1	7	
5	3			2			9	
	1	6	8					5
		9	6				4	

Puzzle 5 (Easy, difficulty rating 0.44)

8			6				3	
			1	9				6
7						2	1	
	7	6		8			9	5
		8		7		6		
1	9			5		7	2	
	3	7						1
9			7	3				
	5				4			7

Puzzle 6 (Easy, difficulty rating 0.40)

				2	9	7		4
	8		4		3			
2	7			1		5		
	5	1						
3		2		5		1		7
						3	6	
		7		9			3	8
			7		4		5	
5			9	6	8			

Puzzle 7 (Easy, difficulty rating 0.45)

		3			8			2
			3			7	1	
	6		5		2	9		8
7						2		
	3		8		7		6	
		9						3
4		5	2		6		8	
	8	1			5			
9			4			3		

Puzzle 8 (Easy, difficulty rating 0.36)

		5	3			6		
			2	6	9	5		4
	9				7			3
				5		3		7
6				2				9
2		4		9				
3			8				5	
5			8	6	7	1		
		2				5	4	

Puzzle 9 (Easy, difficulty rating 0.32)

					2	4	6	9
7				9	8			5
	4			1		7		
6				7		9		
	1						4	
		5		4				6
		2		8			3	
4			6	5				7
3	7	9	1					

Puzzle 10 (Easy, difficulty rating 0.38)

		4						
7		5				4	8	3
		6			3			7
4					7		6	
8		7	3	9	6	1		2
	1			8				5
3			4			9		
9	6	1				3		4
						2		

Puzzle 11 (Easy, difficulty rating 0.44)

	1	2						
		6	8	3			5	
		7	2			4		9
		4			2	3		8
	5						7	
9		8	3			5		
7		5			8	1		
	2			4	6	7		
						9	8	

Puzzle 12 (Easy, difficulty rating 0.35)

3	1					9		
4	9				2			
2	8			1	7	5		
			3			2		
	4		5		9		6	
		9			6			
		1	7	5			8	2
			6				5	7
		3					9	1

Puzzle 13 (Easy, difficulty rating 0.33)

4		7		8	9			
				5		4		7
2						3	1	
3			5	7				
7	4						3	2
				3	8			9
	6	2						3
5		1		6				
			7	2		8		5

Puzzle 14 (Easy, difficulty rating 0.42)

	2	6					8	5
7				5	1		4	3
					8		6	
				4			5	1
			8		5			
5	7		1					
	4		3					
2	6		4	9				8
9	8					7	2	

Puzzle 15 (Easy, difficulty rating 0.43)

	2				1			
		6	9		4	5		8
	7	5				1		
		4	3	9			2	
			1		7			
	9			8	6	3		
		7				9	5	
6		9	4		8	2		
			5				1	

Puzzle 16 (Easy, difficulty rating 0.37)

		1	9		7			
2		3		8			9	4
	9					1		6
8					2		4	
	6			3			1	
	4		5					7
7		6					2	
3	1			6		7		9
			1		3	4		

Puzzle 17 (Easy, difficulty rating 0.42)

	9				8			
						4		3
		6		9	1	2		
	2	3		1		7		6
	5		8		6		2	
6		9		4		5	1	
		7	2	5		8		
9		1						
			1				7	

Puzzle 18 (Easy, difficulty rating 0.30)

7	5						4	9
			8	9			2	1
						6		3
		8	6					5
6	2			5			3	7
3					4	9		
2		4						
1	9			6	3			
5	6						7	4

Puzzle 19 (Easy, difficulty rating 0.28)

4				7	2			6
	9	2		4		3		
8	7						1	
					7		2	
7			2	5	9			8
	1		3					
	6						4	9
		8		3		2	7	
5			9	8				1

Puzzle 20 (Easy, difficulty rating 0.26)

					9	3		
9	7			1	3	2	5	
		6			7		4	
	1							7
8			3		4			2
6							9	
	2		8			7		
	5	9	7	4			6	1
		8	5					

Puzzle 21 (Easy, difficulty rating 0.36)

		1				9	4	
2					3			8
7			9	8		6	1	
					2			9
9	4						5	1
5			7					
	8	6		2	5			7
3			1					4
	7	9				2		

Puzzle 22 (Easy, difficulty rating 0.40)

		7			6			5
		1	5	8				
	9			2	7			6
		1			2		5	3
1								2
3	7		4		5			
9			2	7			6	
			4	9	5			
6			8			1		

Puzzle 23 (Easy, difficulty rating 0.33)

8						9	7	1
5		9	8	3				
	2						3	8
6					7	4		
	8			4			1	
		2	3					7
7	9					8		
			9	4	6			2
2	4	6						3

Puzzle 24 (Easy, difficulty rating 0.35)

2	9	8		4		1		
	5	7			6	9	2	
6					5			
		4	6		2			
				7				
			3			8	6	
			9					2
	4	6	8			3	1	
		2		6		4	7	8

Puzzle 25 (Easy, difficulty rating 0.38)

		3	7	4			2	
		9			3			7
		2			9		3	
	9		6			8		3
		1		7		4		
4		7			8		9	
	7		1			3		
9			8			6		
	1			2	5	7		

Puzzle 26 (Easy, difficulty rating 0.44)

5			4			3		2
	8		1	3	9			5
	4		2					
	9	1	8			2		
		5			6	9	8	
					8		3	
2			6	4	1		5	
8		9			3			4

Puzzle 27 (Easy, difficulty rating 0.37)

		2	6	4			1	5
	8		5	2				
	9				1		8	
					7	2		
	3	9		5		4	7	
		6	3					
	1		9				4	
				1	3		2	
9	4			7	5	8		

Puzzle 28 (Easy, difficulty rating 0.37)

2						9		6
	6	3			5			8
	9	1			3			
9				7			8	
7	1						4	3
	3			1				2
			2			5	6	
5			1			3	2	
1			6					9

Puzzle 29 (Easy, difficulty rating 0.44)

	3	8						6
				1				
	1	7	8				2	3
3	8			9	6		7	2
				3				
4	6		7	8			9	5
1	9				4	5	6	
				6				
8						7	1	

Puzzle 30 (Easy, difficulty rating 0.39)

2			1	5			3	
		5						9
	6			9	4		2	
	3	4			2			1
9								3
1			3			2	9	
	9		8	2			7	
5						8		
	7			3	6			4

Puzzle 31 (Easy, difficulty rating 0.43)

					4		5	3
		3	7					
	4	5		3		1		2
9				7				5
	2		6		9		3	
7				4				6
3		2		6		8	9	
					2	5		
1	9		5					

Puzzle 32 (Easy, difficulty rating 0.42)

		7	4					
9	2		6					
1			7		9	4	3	8
			8	9			4	
6				1				5
	9			6	7			
5	4	9	2		8			7
				6			8	3
				5	2			

Puzzle 33 (Easy, difficulty rating 0.43)

			5		3	8	6	
					1	3		7
2				7	4	5		
8				5				
	6		9		4		2	
			3					9
	4	2	7					5
7		3	6					
	9	5	4		2			

Puzzle 34 (Easy, difficulty rating 0.42)

2					6			
1		6	4		5			
	8		3		1	5		2
					9	6		8
		2		3		9		
7		3	6					
3		1	9		2		8	
			1		3	2		9
			8					4

Puzzle 35 (Easy, difficulty rating 0.44)

	2	5			9			
9		1	8					6
								3
4		8	2		5			7
3	6			1			2	5
1			7		6	4		9
2								
8					1	5		2
			6			1	7	

Puzzle 36 (Easy, difficulty rating 0.36)

6	7			4				5
	2			1			4	6
	5	3	2					7
	9		3					
			1		6			
					2		3	
1					9	4	7	
9	4				3		1	
3					7		5	8

Puzzle 37 (Easy, difficulty rating 0.42)

2	7				1	9		
		4		7				
5	9			3	4			
	5	1		9				2
3								7
6				2		4	9	
			4	8			7	6
				6		2		
		6	2				4	8

Puzzle 38 (Easy, difficulty rating 0.44)

		7				6	1	
							3	4
8			7	1			2	
4	8				1	5		2
			8		5			
9		5	2				7	3
	5			9	3			7
1	2							
	7	9				4		

Puzzle 39 (Easy, difficulty rating 0.42)

3				7		8		
	7	6	8					4
			9	1	6			
6	1					9		
	8	7				1	3	
		9				6	2	
			3	6	1			
4					7	3	2	
		5		4				1

Puzzle 40 (Easy, difficulty rating 0.28)

8					4		1	3
	5			7	6	9		
7		9						
6						3	4	5
2								8
1	3	4						9
						2		4
		7	6	5			9	
9	6		8					7

Puzzle 41 (Easy, difficulty rating 0.35)

		2	8					5
	7			3			4	9
	6	8	4			3	1	
				5			9	
		3				2		
	9			2				
	5	1			2	4	7	
4	3			1			2	
6					3	5		

Puzzle 42 (Easy, difficulty rating 0.42)

2					5		7	
		6	7				9	8
		7	8	3				
	4					3	6	
1	6			4			5	9
	3	8					4	
			7	2	1			
5	2				8	7		
	7		5					4

Puzzle 43 (Easy, difficulty rating 0.42)

	2				1			
3	1		7			9		
	5	8				6	1	
			5	9				4
	6	7		4		2	3	
4				2	6			
	7	5				8	4	
		2			4		9	5
			9				2	

Puzzle 44 (Easy, difficulty rating 0.32)

	5			2	9			
						1	7	
7	9	6				3	2	
			1	5			9	
3	6						2	1
	4		6	9				
		2	8			3	1	4
	1	8						
			2	7			5	

Puzzle 45 (Easy, difficulty rating 0.45)

				5		8		7
7	5			3				
6		3		7		1		
					6	9		2
1	9						8	5
8		6	5					
		1		4		5		6
				8			1	3
5		9		6				

Puzzle 46 (Easy, difficulty rating 0.42)

		8		4	5			
5	1	9			2			
3	7		6			8		
6							9	8
1								4
7	9							6
		1			9		8	2
			1			5	7	9
			2	5		6		

Puzzle 47 (Easy, difficulty rating 0.42)

		6	5		4			
3				2	1	7		9
	2			8			6	
		7	4				9	
5				7				1
	4				6	2		
	7			6			5	
6		5	3	4				8
			8		2	6		

Puzzle 48 (Easy, difficulty rating 0.35)

				8	9			2
3								
	2				5	1	9	4
	9	8			2	4	3	
4				9				7
	7	2	4			5	8	
7	5	4	3				2	
								8
9			7	2				

Puzzle 49 (Easy, difficulty rating 0.36)

3				7			1	6
			8					
	5	4		1				3
	1	3		5				8
	8		6		4		3	
5				3		7	6	
9				6		4	5	
					7			
7	3			4				1

Puzzle 50 (Easy, difficulty rating 0.39)

			7			3	1	
3	9				2			
6			9	3			4	
	8	1	5				2	
		3		7		8		
	2				1	6	9	
	3			4	7			2
		1					7	8
	7	8			9			

MEDIUM

SUDOKU

Puzzle 1 (Medium, difficulty rating 0.56)

		2	4		9			5
4				7	6			
3	6				1			2
		1			4	3		6
			2					
6		5	9			8		
5			8				6	3
			1	6				9
9			3		5	7		

Puzzle 2 (Medium, difficulty rating 0.46)

	7					1		3
		5	3	6				7
				7	8	6		
		3	6				1	
	8	4		1		3	2	
	9				2	5		
		9	7	8				
7				9	3	4		
5		8					7	

Puzzle 3 (Medium, difficulty rating 0.50)

		7		6		3	4	
						2	9	
5			7		4	1		
	2		1				3	8
		6				9		
3	5				8		6	
		8	4		3			1
	7	3						
	1	5		7		8		

Puzzle 4 (Medium, difficulty rating 0.49)

9	1				6			7
	3				1			
4		7	5	2				9
		5				2		
	4		2		7		5	
		1				8		
7				4	2	1		5
			9				2	
1			8				6	3

Puzzle 5 (Medium, difficulty rating 0.52)

1	5		4					
9			6		3			5
					5	9	3	
		1		6	9	8		4
				8				
7		8	1	3		5		
	3	2	9					
5			3		1			8
					6		2	9

Puzzle 6 (Medium, difficulty rating 0.52)

	8	5	7					3
1					6		4	
2		4	9					
	6		5			3	8	
9								7
	5	3			7		1	
				4	7			8
	9		1					6
5					8	9	2	

Puzzle 7 (Medium, difficulty rating 0.59)

		9						
		8	2	5				
4	7	6			8		1	
		7	5	6	9		3	
		3				4		
	6		7	4	3	2		
	9		4			1	7	5
				7	5	9		
						3		

Puzzle 8 (Medium, difficulty rating 0.47)

		8	2		1	9	7	6
7								
3				8				4
	5					8		
8	9		3	5	4		2	1
		2					3	
6				2				7
								8
2	8	5	4		9	1		

Puzzle 9 (Medium, difficulty rating 0.55)

			2					3
	1			6	7		2	
2		8			1			6
7	2	4						1
		6				2		
3						6	8	9
1			5			3		7
	4		6	7			5	
5					2			

Puzzle 10 (Medium, difficulty rating 0.48)

1		9	7			6		8
				1	9			2
		5			8	3		
2		7						1
	9						4	
4						8		5
		6	8			1		
5			9	2				
8		2			3	5		6

Puzzle 11 (Medium, difficulty rating 0.53)

3	4				8			
		7			1	8		
	8	9	5			4	2	
		6				9		3
	2						8	
4		8				2		
	1	2			7	6	4	
		5	8			7		
			1				9	8

Puzzle 12 (Medium, difficulty rating 0.47)

	9		4					
	4		2	1			6	
			8	6		3	5	4
9						7		
	1		3		9		8	
		6						9
7	2	4	6	9				
	3			4	2		9	
				5			1	

Puzzle 13 (Medium, difficulty rating 0.53)

3				1	5		2	
	2		9					4
			6				9	
9	6		3					
	1	5	7		2	9	3	
					9		1	8
	3			6				
5				8		4		
	8		4	5				3

Puzzle 14 (Medium, difficulty rating 0.55)

	3		2	8		4		
5		4		6				7
		2			7		3	
			8					2
	2		4	1	9		7	
4					3			
	1		7			3		
7				3		1		9
		3		9	4		6	

Puzzle 15 (Medium, difficulty rating 0.46)

		4						7
		6	8				5	
				7	9	1		
4		8		2			3	1
	6		7		8		4	
7	1			5		6		2
		2	5	8				
	9				2	8		
8						5		

Puzzle 16 (Medium, difficulty rating 0.60)

6	4		7			9		1
9					5		4	2
			4		8			
		4	6			2		
	1						7	
		9			4	6		
			3		1			
1	6		2					3
3		5			6		2	7

Puzzle 17 (Medium, difficulty rating 0.53)

		1	9				5	2
			2				3	1
	3	9						8
7	2		5	6				
	9			7			6	
				1	2		9	7
3						5	4	
8	6				5			
9	4				1	8		

Puzzle 18 (Medium, difficulty rating 0.48)

7		3		5				
		1		4		5		7
			6	2				8
					6	3	2	
2	9						6	5
	4	6	5					
4				1	5			
5		9		8		2		
				6		8		3

Puzzle 19 (Medium, difficulty rating 0.47)

	2						4	
7				8			9	
9	4	1						5
		4		5	8	1		9
			6		4			
6		8	9	3		7		
5						4	1	6
	8			7				3
	1						7	

Puzzle 20 (Medium, difficulty rating 0.47)

	1	2						4
		8	6		1			9
9	3	5	4				6	
				6				8
	6			5			1	
7			2					
	9				8	7	4	5
3			1		5	9		
8						1	3	

Puzzle 21 (Medium, difficulty rating 0.49)

9			3			2		
	7	1		6				4
	6	8			4			
4	9						1	
	5		6		7		8	
	8						5	6
			4			8	7	
6				2		1	4	
		4			3			9

Puzzle 22 (Medium, difficulty rating 0.46)

	6						5	9
		9	8			1		
	5		9	4				7
		8		9	4			
5	3						9	2
			3	7		5		
9			6	8		3		
		1			7	9		
7	4						6	

Puzzle 23 (Medium, difficulty rating 0.46)

2		1	8					
	4					8	9	3
				7			1	
4	6	2	9					
	7	8				1	5	
					3	6	4	2
	2			5				
5	1	3					2	
					6	4		5

Puzzle 24 (Medium, difficulty rating 0.52)

	5				9	7		6
	2	1	3					4
			1				2	3
	3			8			6	
9			2					8
	4		6				7	
3	1			9				
7					6	2	4	
5		2	8				3	

Puzzle 25 (Medium, difficulty rating 0.54)

8	4	2	6					7
	3	6		4				
	9		2					
					6			1
	5	8	3		2	7	4	
4			5					
					4		7	
				8		1	6	
7					3	2	9	4

Puzzle 26 (Medium, difficulty rating 0.52)

				2	6		9	3
					7	2		
7	6		3			4	1	
5	3							7
	2						8	
8							6	9
	9	4			3		7	2
	6	7						
2	7		9	6				

Puzzle 27 (Medium, difficulty rating 0.56)

2			1	5		7		4
		4		9	6	5		
6			9		1		5	
3		2				8		9
	1		8		2			3
		3	6	7		9		
4		9		2	5			7

Puzzle 28 (Medium, difficulty rating 0.53)

	7	1	6	9			4	
			2		4			
8			5		7			9
7	8							1
		5		4		7		
3							9	2
1			9		6			4
			8		2			
	2			3	1	9	5	

Puzzle 29 (Medium, difficulty rating 0.48)

9	6		2					8
			7			2	6	
		4			3	7		
		9			7	6		1
6				4				3
5		1	3			8		
		5	4			9		
	4	6			8			
8					6		4	2

Puzzle 30 (Medium, difficulty rating 0.59)

	6	5		2	1	7	8	3
	3						4	
1				4	5			
			6					7
			2	1	8			
6				9				
		6	4					8
	8						3	
2	1	3	8	5		6	9	

Puzzle 31 (Medium, difficulty rating 0.59)

	5			2	1		4	
2								5
		4		8	5		6	
7	9			4	3	8		
		5	9	7			1	4
	7		8	5		6		
5								2
	8		2	6			5	

Puzzle 32 (Medium, difficulty rating 0.58)

7			4		6	1		
6					5	9		
	9			8				4
2			1		9	6		
	5						4	
		6	5		4			2
5				2			3	
		1	3					5
		3	9		7			6

Puzzle 33 (Medium, difficulty rating 0.46)

	4			7				
			6	8		5		
8			2			7	1	
		2		4	7		6	8
			9		2			
5	8		3	1		9		
	7	1			9			5
	9		8	2				
			5				3	

Puzzle 34 (Medium, difficulty rating 0.56)

			9				2	
2	3					8		
	7	4		5	2		3	
			8	9	3			
	5	6		4		1	9	
		2	3	1				
	8		4	2		9	1	
		1					4	5
	4				1			

Puzzle 35 (Medium, difficulty rating 0.54)

1		2				9		
5				9			6	
	9	3			6			1
3			4	7	8			
		8				7		
			2	3	5			6
6			5			8	1	
	1			2				7
		5				6		2

Puzzle 36 (Medium, difficulty rating 0.47)

		6						2
8	5		2		4	9		
			5			3		
	4		6		2			
2	6		3		8		5	4
			7		1		9	
		2			3			
	8	4		7			2	3
4						6		

27

Puzzle 37 (Medium, difficulty rating 0.59)

	9	7	8			3	4	
						1		8
6				3		2		
1			5			4		
4	7						8	9
		2			9			7
	2			9				4
7		6						
	4	1			2	8	6	

Puzzle 38 (Medium, difficulty rating 0.56)

					9	7	4	
		1				8		5
	4		5	7				
4				6				
7	8	9	2		1	3	5	6
				3				7
			1	8			6	
8		4				9		
	3	6	7					

Puzzle 39 (Medium, difficulty rating 0.51)

					9		5	4
1			7				6	
		2		6		8		1
8			9				4	
		3	5		2	1		
	1				6			5
4		6		9		2	.	
	5				7			9
3	9		2					

Puzzle 40 (Medium, difficulty rating 0.47)

4	9	7		5				
	8	5	2			9		
				7			8	
	5	2	8		4			3
				2				
1			6			3	2	7
	1			6				
		9			1	8	5	
				8		4	6	1

Puzzle 41 (Medium, difficulty rating 0.60)

			2			7	9	
			1	7	4	2		8
6			3					
	9	5			8			
8	4			3			2	5
			5			4	8	
					1			2
1		8	6	2	3			
	6	2			5			

Puzzle 42 (Medium, difficulty rating 0.50)

		3	8			6	5	
		5		6	4			
	4				9	1		
			1	9		2	4	6
				2				
2	8	1		4	7			
		4	2				1	
			9	3		4		
	1	9			6	7		

Puzzle 43 (Medium, difficulty rating 0.53)

	5	1	4				9	6
6				2				5
		7			6	4		
				9	3			
	7	9		6			1	5
			1	5				
		4	7			6		
8				1				4
7	6				2	8	1	

Puzzle 44 (Medium, difficulty rating 0.56)

8			4	5			1	
						5		4
	2	5		4			8	
5						8	2	
		1	8	5	2	7		
	8	3						9
	9			3		1	4	
1			8					
	5				9	6		7

Puzzle 45 (Medium, difficulty rating 0.57)

	7		8	1		2		4
	9			3				
4		2			7	1		
2					1			
	4		3		2		7	
			5					2
		3	4			9		7
				7			6	
5		7		2	8		3	

Puzzle 46 (Medium, difficulty rating 0.54)

1			5			2		
8	2		4					3
6				3				2
5	7	2					8	
		6				7		
	9					4	1	5
7			2					8
2					4		9	1
			8		5			7

Puzzle 47 (Medium, difficulty rating 0.60)

				5				
4	3	6					9	
5	2					4	1	
			1		5	9	6	
	8	5				3	7	
	9	2	7		6			
	6	8					4	7
	7					2	5	9
				1				

Puzzle 48 (Medium, difficulty rating 0.47)

		1	9	8				
	7	9	6				3	
3							2	
8	9					3	5	
7			8		2			9
	6	3					7	8
	8							3
	4				8	2	9	
				7	1	6		

Puzzle 49 (Medium, difficulty rating 0.54)

			1					
8			3	9	7		5	
7	3			6			4	
	4		9					1
	9	8				6	3	
1					6		9	
	7			4			8	2
	2		8	1	9			5
					3			

Puzzle 50 (Medium, difficulty rating 0.56)

5	4		8	1		6	7	
8								
1			9					
7					6		8	
4		8	7	3	2	9		6
	9		1					7
					5			2
								1
	2	7		8	1		4	5

HARD
SUDOKU

Puzzle 1 (Hard, difficulty rating 0.66)

	8		9		3			5
			4			2	9	
		5			7	3		
	4	3				9		7
			3		6			
9		8				6	1	
		6	2			8		
	3	9			1			
7			6		9		3	

Puzzle 2 (Hard, difficulty rating 0.69)

		8	1	7				
		2					7	3
			2	4	3			9
	1	9		5		3		
7								6
		3		1		5	4	
5			4	3	8			
8	2					4		
				2	1	8		

Puzzle 3 (Hard, difficulty rating 0.65)

		5	2					7
							4	1
7	6				8	3	2	5
			4		2		1	3
				8				
3	1		7		5			
4	3	2	8				5	6
5	8							
6					1	4		

Puzzle 4 (Hard, difficulty rating 0.62)

1	7	3	5			2		
	4	5			3			
				2				5
	6	1					4	
3		2		8		6		7
	5					1	8	
5				9				
			3			8	2	
		8			7	5	9	6

Puzzle 5 (Hard, difficulty rating 0.71)

5	8			7	6		2	
				9	4			
		3	5		4		7	
8	3	2				9		
		6				8	4	2
	2		4		5	7		
		8	9					
	1		7	3			9	6

Puzzle 6 (Hard, difficulty rating 0.67)

7				1	4			
		1	9		2			
	9			3	8			1
		3			5		9	8
		5		7		1		
2	8		1			3		
8			3	6			1	
			4			1	5	
			5	2				4

Puzzle 7 (Hard, difficulty rating 0.66)

				1			7	2
	7		8				6	
5		4		7	8			
	4			8		1		6
	1						2	
8		3		9			4	
		7	3			2		9
	8				4		1	
1	9			2				

Puzzle 8 (Hard, difficulty rating 0.74)

2	1				5		3	
	6			9		8		
7			6					
		3	5	4	9		8	
		1				5		
	5		3	8	1	4		
				6				9
	6		5				4	
	3		9				5	6

Puzzle 9 (Hard, difficulty rating 0.61)

		5						
9		4				3	5	
			5	4	1		6	
3		8	4					6
	5		3		2		7	
4					6	1		5
	4		2	6	7			
	8	9				6		7
						4		

Puzzle 10 (Hard, difficulty rating 0.60)

	9		4			8	1	6
					3			
		4			6	2		3
	1	3			2		4	
2								5
	4		1			7	6	
9		8	3			4		
			5					
7	3	5			9		8	

Puzzle 11 (Hard, difficulty rating 0.74)

	8	7		1	5			3
	9			3		6		
1			9					5
	5			9			7	6
8	4			5			2	
6					2			9
	7		4				1	
9			5	6		3	8	

Puzzle 12 (Hard, difficulty rating 0.65)

4	1						9	2
9		3		6	4			
			9			3		
2			6		8			
	9	6		4		8	2	
			5		9			6
		9			2			
			3	8		9		4
1	8						7	3

Puzzle 13 (Hard, difficulty rating 0.63)

```
. 9 8 | . . . | . . 2
. 3 5 | 4 9 2 | . . .
. . . | . . 1 | 9 . .
------+-------+------
. . . | 1 . . | . . 7
9 8 7 | . . . | 3 1 5
5 . . | . 7 . | . . .
------+-------+------
. . 4 | 9 . . | . . .
. . 7 | 6 5 4 | 2 . .
2 . . | . . . | 7 9 .
```

Puzzle 14 (Hard, difficulty rating 0.63)

```
. . . | . . 4 | 7 3 .
3 5 7 | 9 . . | . 4 .
9 . 4 | 3 . . | . . .
------+-------+------
. . 2 | 4 . . | . . .
. 3 . | 8 . 2 | . 6 .
. . . | . . 9 | 4 . .
------+-------+------
. . . | . . . | 5 8 6
. 8 . | . . 3 | 2 5 4
. 2 5 | 1 . . | . . .
```

Puzzle 15 (Hard, difficulty rating 0.70)

```
. 7 3 | . . 8 | . 4 9
. . . | . . . | 5 . 8
6 . . | . 5 . | . . .
------+-------+------
. . . | 5 . . | 1 3 .
7 9 5 | . . . | 4 2 6
. 6 1 | . . 2 | . . .
------+-------+------
. . . | . 4 . | . . 2
9 . 6 | . . . | . . .
2 3 . | 1 . . | 7 9 .
```

Puzzle 16 (Hard, difficulty rating 0.70)

```
. 1 . | . . . | 6 3 .
7 . . | 2 . 8 | . . .
. . . | . . . | . 4 2
------+-------+------
. . 9 | . 5 . | 8 . 3
1 2 . | 4 3 7 | . 6 5
3 . 6 | . 8 . | 2 . .
------+-------+------
9 8 . | . . . | . . .
. . . | 8 . 4 | . . 7
. 4 7 | . . . | . 8 .
```

Puzzle 17 (Hard, difficulty rating 0.62)

9								8
3				5			6	
						4	9	5
	8		3	7	1	2	5	
			2	4	8			
	3	2	5	6	9		7	
6	2	4						
	5			3				1
8								7

Puzzle 18 (Hard, difficulty rating 0.67)

							5	
4		2	1		5		8	6
			8	7	3			2
	8	6						1
	9					3		
7						6	9	
8		9	5	7				
2	1		6		4	8		5
	4							

Puzzle 19 (Hard, difficulty rating 0.64)

	8	7			9		6	
	6		8				2	
		2		3	1		4	7
						3	9	1
8	2	1						
4	3		1	6		2		
	1				5		3	
	5		3			6	1	

Puzzle 20 (Hard, difficulty rating 0.64)

				8				
				9	4	2		6
			3	2		9	5	
9		1		7				2
	3		2		8		9	
2				6		4		3
	2	8		5	7			
3		6	4	1				
				3				

Puzzle 21 (Hard, difficulty rating 0.70)

7	4			8	3			
		8	2	9				7
	3	9					6	
		6	9					
	2	3				1	9	
					2	4		
	6					5	4	
3				2	9	6		
			5	1			8	3

Puzzle 22 (Hard, difficulty rating 0.64)

9				2	7			8
			6		1	9	7	
							1	2
				4	1	2		
3	5						4	6
	1	2	7					
8	9							
	2	6	4		5			
7			1	9				5

Puzzle 23 (Hard, difficulty rating 0.61)

			2				6	
		7			8		9	
9	1			6		4		
3			1			8		
	9	4	7		3	6	5	
		2			6			9
		6		4			3	5
	3		6			7		
	4				5			

Puzzle 24 (Hard, difficulty rating 0.60)

		8	7				2	
4	7		2		8			1
2				9	4			
		7	8					6
6				9				7
9				2	8			
		3	1					9
8			3		4		5	2
	6			7	1			

Puzzle 25 (Hard, difficulty rating 0.60)

		8		3	5		1	
		9						
	4			6	2	3		
	7	5	2	4				1
4								6
2				7	1	9	4	
		4	5	9			7	
						5		
	9		4	2		1		

Puzzle 26 (Hard, difficulty rating 0.71)

			9		6		1	
6	3		4		5	9	7	
	5							
2					1	7	8	
	8						6	
	1	9	8					5
							9	
	9	3	2		8		5	1
	2		7		9			

Puzzle 27 (Hard, difficulty rating 0.64)

		4				7	2	
				4				1
6	9	7		2		8		3
	1		4		3			9
7			1		6		5	
8		1		5		4	3	7
5				3				
	7	3				5		

Puzzle 28 (Hard, difficulty rating 0.63)

5		7					2	
	4	3		5				7
	2							5
7	9			3	4			
4			2	7	1			9
			5	9			3	4
3							6	
6				2		1	7	
	1					9		8

Puzzle 29 (Hard, difficulty rating 0.60)

	5				8		9	
	1			2			4	5
6			4					1
				3		2		
9	2		5		1		3	4
		8		6				
5					3			2
2	7			5			8	
	9		6				1	

Puzzle 30 (Hard, difficulty rating 0.67)

4						7	6	1
7	2			1				
	6				5			2
	4	8			7		3	
			5		4			
	5		2			9	8	
5			3				7	
				5			4	3
6	1	3						9

Puzzle 31 (Hard, difficulty rating 0.70)

		7	5				9	
	3	2	6				1	
9	8			4	3			
		4			2	9		5
2		3	9			1		
			4	6			2	8
	2				7	6	4	
	4				5	3		

Puzzle 32 (Hard, difficulty rating 0.60)

		4		7		5		
8					1			
	6			2	3			
7	9	3				8		2
6	8						7	1
4		1				3	6	5
			5	9			1	
			7					9
		8		1		2		

Puzzle 33 (Hard, difficulty rating 0.65)

	4		3					9
	5	2				8		
3	9			2				
	6				8	9	1	4
		4				3		
9	8	3	4				6	
				8			9	7
		9				1	2	
1					7		5	

Puzzle 34 (Hard, difficulty rating 0.61)

		8			1			
	4				6	5		
		1		5		3	9	6
		3					5	7
	2	6				9	8	
4	9					6		
9	3	2		1		7		
		5	4				3	
			3			1		

Puzzle 35 (Hard, difficulty rating 0.70)

					4		3	
					2	1		7
9	7		5	3				
			8	4			1	6
6		1				4		8
8	5			6	9			
				1	8		7	5
2		6	3					
	1		4					

Puzzle 36 (Hard, difficulty rating 0.62)

	6		5		1			
	2				7	9	1	
	3			2	4			6
			1	7			9	
		2				7		
	7			4	8			
3			7	1			2	
	9	1	4				8	
			8		5		6	

Puzzle 37 (Hard, difficulty rating 0.61)

	1				8			5
8							3	7
3	9	6			4		2	
5			2			7		
	3						1	
		7		6				8
	7		4			1	8	9
1	2							6
4			9			7		

Puzzle 38 (Hard, difficulty rating 0.64)

			4	2				
	7		1				8	6
	5			8	7	3		
		6	7	4		5		
	9						3	
		4		5	1	6		
		9	5	7			1	
2	1				4		7	
				1	3			

Puzzle 39 (Hard, difficulty rating 0.60)

		3	6	8			9	
						6		1
	6		1		3		8	
9	5				1			
4		1				2		9
			9				4	8
	1		3		8		2	
2		8						
	3			1	4	8		

Puzzle 40 (Hard, difficulty rating 0.66)

6				1			3	
					8	7	2	
	1			5	8			
9	2	1						8
	8		4		9		1	
4						9	7	2
		3	5				9	
	9	7	3					
	6			9				4

Puzzle 41 (Hard, difficulty rating 0.61)

	8		5	1			3	
		3			7	9		8
	9				3			
6			2		4			1
	5						2	
1			9		8			5
			7				8	
7		1	8			2		
	2			9	1		5	

Puzzle 42 (Hard, difficulty rating 0.70)

					1		8	
5		9			4			
8			9		3	7		
1	2	5					4	9
3								1
6	8					3	7	2
		1	3		2			7
			5			2		8
	6		7					

Puzzle 43 (Hard, difficulty rating 0.65)

3	7		9				8	1
		9						2
5			8			4	7	
	3			1	5			
			3		4			
			2	7			1	
	9	1			8			5
6						1		
7	5				1		9	8

Puzzle 44 (Hard, difficulty rating 0.68)

	4	8	6					3
	3		5					
5	7				3	6		
				4		3	6	5
		5		7		8		
6	9	3	2					
		7	8				4	2
					1		8	
8					2	9	3	

43

Puzzle 45 (Hard, difficulty rating 0.75)

7		9					8	
			3			9		
		5			7	3	2	
3	5	1		2				9
			3	9	6			
6				4		2	3	8
	7	2	4			8		
		3		1				
	4					1		3

Puzzle 46 (Hard, difficulty rating 0.63)

4	6				1	7		3
			7				4	
				8		5		
9	2						5	
3		7	2		8	4		9
	4						1	2
		6		3				
	8				6			
2		3	8				9	4

Puzzle 47 (Hard, difficulty rating 0.60)

				3				
				6	8		5	
	8	6	7			9		
	5	1					9	
8	4	9	3		5	2	7	6
	3					1	8	
		7			6	3	1	
	9		5	2				
				4				

Puzzle 48 (Hard, difficulty rating 0.63)

	8			4		1		
			5	9	6			4
	1						7	5
			3	2	5			1
2								3
1			8	9	6			
5	9						1	
7		2	9	3				
		1		7			9	

Puzzle 49 (Hard, difficulty rating 0.66)

	7		3					5
		9	6				3	
	2	6			1			7
	1	7		8			2	6
9	4			2		1	7	
1			7			5	8	
	9				8	7		
7				9			4	

Puzzle 50 (Hard, difficulty rating 0.63)

		1		4		2	8	5
			5				4	
		3		6	8			7
2						7	6	
			1		6			
	1	6						4
1			6	2		4		
	4				5			
3	6	2		7		9		

VERY HARD

SUDOKU

Puzzle 1 (Very hard, difficulty rating 0.76)

7				8			2	
		6					7	
8				3	7	1		9
	3		8					5
		1	3	7	6	2		
2					5		3	
4		3	2	1				7
	2					9		
	8			5				2

Puzzle 2 (Very hard, difficulty rating 0.80)

4						9		3
		2			3		1	6
	7		6		9		2	
8	9	3						
		7		4		8		
						3	7	1
	3		7		2		4	
1	4		5			2		
7		8						5

Puzzle 3 (Very hard, difficulty rating 0.78)

2						8	3	
		9	1	2			4	
		7	6			5		
	7			4				8
		4	3		1	2		
1				8			6	
		8			3	1		
	9			5	2	4		
	4	2						3

Puzzle 4 (Very hard, difficulty rating 0.78)

	2				3	9		
	8			6			3	
			8				6	4
			1		8	3		
	6	7	5		2	4	1	
		4	7		6			
6	4				1			
	9			5			4	
		3	6				5	

Puzzle 5 (Very hard, difficulty rating 0.77)

9	3					2		
			3	4		6	1	
		6						3
1			4		9	3	2	8
4	8	9	2		3			1
2						1		
	4	1		9	7			
		8					9	5

Puzzle 6 (Very hard, difficulty rating 0.85)

8								4
				1	7	2		
6			8	4		3	7	
2		8		3	9			
	6						8	
			4	8		1		3
	7	2		6	4			5
		3	5	9				
5								1

Puzzle 7 (Very hard, difficulty rating 0.77)

				7			4	
		8	4				1	
	4		6	9				7
		9		5				8
4		3	7		8	9		1
1				3		7		
3				8	7		2	
	5				6	1		
	6			1				

Puzzle 8 (Very hard, difficulty rating 0.79)

			1	6	5			7
	1	4						
	8		7			4		1
	2			4		5		
		9	2			1	6	
		8		5				1
2			4			7		6
						1	2	
4			3	1	2			

Puzzle 9 (Very hard, difficulty rating 0.80)

6	2		7		1			9
			2		6	1		5
		6		1		9		
9	5		4	7	8		2	6
		4		6		5		
7		8	5		4			
5			6		7		9	4

Puzzle 10 (Very hard, difficulty rating 0.75)

3					9			
	5				8		9	6
	8	9	7	4			3	
	4		8					
5		7		1		8		9
				2			7	
	9			8	3	1	5	
8	7		4				6	
			5					8

Puzzle 11 (Very hard, difficulty rating 0.83)

5							2	7
9					4		8	
		6		1	2			4
				5	8	4	6	
			4		6			
	6	9	7	3				
3			6	4		8		
	8		1					6
6	9							5

Puzzle 12 (Very hard, difficulty rating 0.84)

6	9	8				3		
4		1			8		2	5
			4			8		
			3			2	6	
	1						8	
	2	5			6			
		7		9				
1	6		5			9		8
		4				1	5	2

Puzzle 13 (Very hard, difficulty rating 0.90)

3			4			1		
6	2					4	9	
	8	4				7		6
	5			2	9			
			8		3			
			7	5			1	
5		3				2	7	
	4	8					3	1
		2			7			8

Puzzle 14 (Very hard, difficulty rating 0.96)

		4						
	3	6	8		5		2	
8	2		7		6			
		3			7		6	1
			1	5	3			
9	1		4			3		
			5			2	8	4
	5		6		4	2	1	
						7		

Puzzle 15 (Very hard, difficulty rating 0.76)

1	7					3		
			4		3		1	
4		3	6		1	2		
	9				4			
5	4			9			2	1
			7				9	
		9	1		5	6		8
	6		2		7			
		4					3	2

Puzzle 16 (Very hard, difficulty rating 0.81)

		8		7			1	
	7	3		2			8	
			8	9	1			
2				6				5
	4	9		3		1		
6				8				4
			7	3	9			
	3		5			6	9	
	4			1		5		

Puzzle 17 (Very hard, difficulty rating 0.91)

	9	6			2	8		
2			8					
8					4	6		2
		2				5		7
	6	4				9	2	
7		8				4		
6		7	9					4
					8			5
		5	3			7	9	

Puzzle 18 (Very hard, difficulty rating 0.81)

9	2		6			1	5	
7					1			
		6	5		8			3
		5	7				1	
	8						3	
	6				3	4		
5			3		6	7		
			1					2
	7	1			2		9	6

Puzzle 19 (Very hard, difficulty rating 0.83)

							2	7
		1			3			5
	2		6	5	9	8		
				1	5		4	
		5	9	4	2	6		
	4		3	6				
		4	5	9	6		8	
9				4			1	
5	7							

Puzzle 20 (Very hard, difficulty rating 0.98)

			3			1		6
					9	2	5	4
				1		3	9	
		4	2	9				
	1		7		8		6	
				5	6	9		
	4	5		8				
1	7	8	9					
2		6			7			

Puzzle 21 (Very hard, difficulty rating 0.84)

	7						2	
2		4	6	1	9			
3					5	4		
4	6		9					1
			5		7			
5					1		3	2
		5	1					3
			3	9	2	5		6
	3						9	

Puzzle 22 (Very hard, difficulty rating 0.87)

7	4		8	9				3
6	8			4		1		
		5						
5		9		3	2			
	6						7	
			4	6		9		5
						8		
		6		8			1	7
8				1	3		4	6

Puzzle 23 (Very hard, difficulty rating 0.90)

			4				5	8
	3				7		9	
1						4		
		2	5		4		7	6
		4	6		2	5		
5	6		3		8	9		
		3						5
	5		2			3		
9	2				5			

Puzzle 24 (Very hard, difficulty rating 0.79)

	3		8	2		5		
	7			6				
2	5	8	9				1	
	8					6		
5			6		9			4
		6					2	
	4				7	1	6	5
				9			4	
		2		4	6		3	

Puzzle 25 (Very hard, difficulty rating 0.82)

9	6			4		1		
			3	8				
7		8		6				9
1	2		8			9		3
				5				
3		5			2		6	4
8				9		4		7
				3	8			
		9		2			8	5

Puzzle 26 (Very hard, difficulty rating 0.82)

			9		1	7		3
				8			1	
			7	5	9			
5	8		3			1	2	
4								5
	2	7			9		4	6
		1	8	9				
	3		7					
9		8	5		4			

Puzzle 27 (Very hard, difficulty rating 0.93)

9	8	5	3					
7				8		9		
	1			9	7		3	
8		6						
2			4		8			5
						3		9
	9		6	4			1	
		1		7				3
					1	6	9	4

Puzzle 28 (Very hard, difficulty rating 0.86)

	8	6			3			4
1						2	7	
	4				1	3	6	
			3	1	4			
		1				9		
			5	9	2			
	6	9	7				2	
	1	5						6
8			1			7	5	

Puzzle 29 (Very hard, difficulty rating 0.79)

		4				3		9
				3		6	1	
5	6	3	9					
4						1	5	
1		7		6		9		2
	2	9						7
					3	8	2	1
	4	1		8				
2		8				5		

Puzzle 30 (Very hard, difficulty rating 0.83)

2					7			9
	3		2	1			8	7
		8			4			
					8		5	2
5		9		7		8		4
8	6		4					
			5			7		
4	9			8	6		2	
3			1					5

Puzzle 31 (Very hard, difficulty rating 0.80)

	1		6		5			8
8			4				6	7
6				8				
5		2				4		
4	6						7	2
	7					5		1
				6				5
9	5				8			4
2			5		1		3	

Puzzle 32 (Very hard, difficulty rating 0.90)

		1	2	9		6	3	
		7	6		8		2	
		2			4			5
	5							3
		6				9		
8							4	
6			4			3		
	9		7			1	2	
	2	5		6	3	4		

Puzzle 33 (Very hard, difficulty rating 0.87)

2			7	8				
1	3		4		5	8	9	
					1	5		
				7			3	
	6		5		4		7	
	9			1				
		1	9					
	7	8	1		3		5	9
				6	7			4

Puzzle 34 (Very hard, difficulty rating 0.79)

	1		9					
			2		1		3	
3		7			4		1	
5		4				1		
6	3		8	1	5		4	2
		1				3		6
	9		3			4		1
	6		4		8			
				6		2		

Puzzle 35 (Very hard, difficulty rating 0.84)

								8
5		3					6	
9	2		3			4		5
		6	9				5	
8	9		5		2		4	1
	5				7	8		
6		4			5		1	3
	3					5		4
2								

Puzzle 36 (Very hard, difficulty rating 0.83)

1								
	5				7		6	1
6			8	1			3	
5	1	7			2		4	8
				5				
9	2		4			7	1	5
	3			8	5			6
8	9		6				7	
								3

Puzzle 37 (Very hard, difficulty rating 0.75)

	1	9	2		6			8
6							2	
	3				1	5		
	9			3	5		6	
		6				4		
	5		8	6			1	
		3	7				5	
	4							2
7			5		4	1	9	

Puzzle 38 (Very hard, difficulty rating 0.76)

	2			3		1		7
7			9					4
4				7	8			
3	4					2		8
		7				6		
2		9					7	5
			3	8				1
6					7			2
8		1		5			9	

Puzzle 39 (Very hard, difficulty rating 0.79)

	4				5		3	8
2						6		
6	8	3	7					
	5	1	9	8				4
4				7	2	3	9	
					7	5	8	6
		2						3
5	7		4				1	

Puzzle 40 (Very hard, difficulty rating 0.80)

	8	2				6		4
7	9			4	1	5		
				8				
		8		2		1	6	3
3	7	6		1		4		
				3				
		5	8	6			7	1
2		7				8	3	

Puzzle 41 (Very hard, difficulty rating 0.84)

7			5			8		
1	2	3	7			5		
		8			6		3	1
4			1		2			
			9		4			2
2	3		6			4		
		5			7	1	8	3
		1			5			6

Puzzle 42 (Very hard, difficulty rating 0.88)

						1		6
			2	3			7	
7			4		9			8
6	9					7		1
	5	1		6		8	9	
3		7					6	5
8			1		4			2
	3			5	8			
1		5						

Puzzle 43 (Very hard, difficulty rating 0.81)

						6	4	
3	9				4	2	8	
				3			7	9
					7		1	8
		2	9		8	7		
7	4		6					
9	8			7				
	7	3	1				9	5
	1	4						

Puzzle 44 (Very hard, difficulty rating 0.80)

			1	2			4	7
2							6	
		3	5		7	1		9
1		5		9	8			
			3	2		5		6
8		1	2		6	9		
	7							1
9	5		1	4				

Puzzle 45 (Very hard, difficulty rating 0.80)

4	3						2	5
		2	5			6		
			9		3			
		3		4	5			8
2		4				7		6
9			6	1		5		
			4		8			
		6			7	4		
8	4						5	7

Puzzle 46 (Very hard, difficulty rating 0.78)

		7				2		
		9	2		5			
		8	6	7		9		4
	1	5	8					6
8				3				9
9					1	7	8	
3		6		2	9	8		
			3			8	6	
		2				5		

Puzzle 47 (Very hard, difficulty rating 0.80)

	6				3		2	
					1		8	6
5		1				4		
			6	9			4	
6	4	3		1		8	5	9
	5			4	8			
		5				3		4
2	7		1					
	8		5				1	

Puzzle 48 (Very hard, difficulty rating 0.81)

3		4						
	2		1		3			
	7					8		3
	8		3		5		9	
	3	9	2		7	5	6	
	5		9		6		8	
2		7					3	
			6		9		2	
						6		1

Puzzle 49 (Very hard, difficulty rating 0.80)

					9	3	5	
		3	8	5			2	4
	5		2					
3					6	4		
	9	4		3			1	8
		1	9					3
					4		3	
2	4			9	8	7		
	3	9	7					

Puzzle 50 (Very hard, difficulty rating 0.79)

	4		3					
	7	1	8			5		
2	6	8	5			7	3	
					5	3		
	5			4			8	
		2	1					
	2	9			6	8	7	3
		7			8	1	4	
					3		2	

RANDOM

SUDOKU

Puzzle 1 (Hard, difficulty rating 0.73)

9	7				1			4
5	4			3				
1			9		4	8		
	8		1					
6		1				7		8
					7		4	
		5	3		6			2
				9			3	7
3			4				8	5

Puzzle 2 (Easy, difficulty rating 0.36)

5			4	1	6			
9				2	8	4		
1							3	
	3		1		7		6	
	5			4			1	
	6		9		5		7	
	1							3
		8	5	7				6
			8	6	1			5

Puzzle 3 (Hard, difficulty rating 0.67)

			4			2		1
5			2				6	
2	7	1		8	6			4
	5						4	3
				2				
3	8					2		
7			6	9		8	3	5
	3				2			7
8		9			5			

Puzzle 4 (Easy, difficulty rating 0.37)

		8	9			2		
9		7			1			
	3		6		8		9	
8	2			6				
3			7		5			8
			3				6	1
	9		5		4		3	
			1			7		2
		2			7	9		

Puzzle 5 (Medium, difficulty rating 0.52)

			3	1		4		9
								3
3	1	9				6	2	5
4					9	8		
		1		2		3		
		6	8					2
6	3	7				1	5	8
8								
1		2		8	7			

Puzzle 6 (Easy, difficulty rating 0.21)

3		8	7		4			
	7							
	2	9	6			8	7	
	3			1			9	4
		5		4		6		
8	6			2			1	
	9	7			3	4	2	
							5	
			9		8	7		6

Puzzle 7 (Hard, difficulty rating 0.61)

3	4						7	
		7	1		4		6	
				2	7	4		
	6				9			3
	7		2		8		1	
4			3				9	
		2	8	7				
	9		6		3	1		
	8						5	7

Puzzle 8 (Medium, difficulty rating 0.49)

			4	2		9	3	
1			5	6	8	4		
	3							
7		1	2					
9	2		1			6	7	
			6			2		9
						5		
	9	2	1	7				6
5	4		6	3				

Puzzle 9 (Very hard, difficulty rating 0.77)

				2		7	9	
			4			6		
6					1		2	5
	7		2	5				9
5	1						7	2
8				1	7		3	
3	8		1					6
		1			2			
	5	6		4				

Puzzle 10 (Medium, difficulty rating 0.48)

	9	3	6	5	7		8	
	1	8	2	4		6		
							9	
	8							1
			8	2	6			
7							6	
	3							
		4		6	1	9	5	
	6		4	8	5	2	3	

Puzzle 11 (Easy, difficulty rating 0.43)

5	9					4		2
			6		9	1		
					4			6
3	5			6	8	2		
	8						4	
		7	1	4			5	8
6			8					
		2	3		7			
7		5					8	9

Puzzle 12 (Easy, difficulty rating 0.34)

			5			3		
	5			1		9	8	2
9		7			2			4
				8		1	2	
	4			9			6	
	2	3		5				
1			3			7		9
3	7	4		2		6		
		6			8			

Puzzle 13 (Easy, difficulty rating 0.37)

8		7	1				9	4
6						8	3	2
	3		4	6				
			7					
		3	5		6	4		
				9				
				7	2		4	
2	4	1						3
7	9				4	5		6

Puzzle 14 (Hard, difficulty rating 0.61)

		6					4	
9	8				2		1	
	2		3		4	6		8
	9			3	6			
			5		1			
			7	8			6	
4		8	1		5		9	
	7		9				8	6
	5					1		

Puzzle 15 (Very hard, difficulty rating 0.83)

						5		9
	5				6	2	3	
2			3	5			7	
	8	4	7				6	5
7	9				8	4	1	
	7			8	1			2
	2	9	4				5	
8			6					

Puzzle 16 (Hard, difficulty rating 0.69)

					8		3	
	6					9		
3		8		4	9	7	6	
8						6	7	
	3	6				8	5	
	7	5						3
	9	7	2	1		4		5
		4					1	
	5		8					

Puzzle 17 (Medium, difficulty rating 0.52)

1			7		9	2		8
			3	6				4
3						9		
			2	9				
9		6	1		7	4		2
				4	6			
		7						1
8				1	2			
4		2	9		8			5

Puzzle 18 (Hard, difficulty rating 0.67)

5						4	3	2
4	2				9			
1		3	2		4			
							1	7
		1	5		2	6		
2	6							
			8		5	7		4
			3				6	1
7	1	5						9

Puzzle 19 (Very hard, difficulty rating 0.89)

							6	
	7		8		1		9	
			7		3		1	4
	4	2	5				8	
7			2		8			5
	8				7	6	2	
8	3		6		2			
	2		3		4		5	
	9							

Puzzle 20 (Medium, difficulty rating 0.56)

	2							
3		9	6				5	2
	7		9			4		
2		8			6		3	1
6								4
7	9		5			6		8
		4			8		1	
8	5				1	3		6
							4	

Puzzle 21 (Easy, difficulty rating 0.43)

						8		6
9				6	8		7	1
		7						
		9		3	5	1		2
6		3				5		9
1		4	6	9		3		
						6		
4	1		7	8				3
2		5						

Puzzle 22 (Easy, difficulty rating 0.44)

		4			3			5
	7	1	9			8		
5	3						1	4
	5	3		8				
	6			7			3	
				5		1	8	
9	4						6	8
		6			4	7	5	
7			2			4		

Puzzle 23 (Medium, difficulty rating 0.47)

2					7			
5	6			1		8		2
			2			3	6	
	2	7			1			3
4				3				8
3			7			5	4	
	5	3			2			
9		2		5			8	6
			6					5

Puzzle 24 (Easy, difficulty rating 0.43)

			7					5
		7			4			8
5			1		8		9	
4	1		2				3	
	9		4		3		2	
	3				5		8	7
	2		5		1			3
8			6			1		
3				7				

Puzzle 25 (Easy, difficulty rating 0.41)

	4	5			2	7		9
			5		4			2
6	1		9					
8					5			6
			8	2	3			
2			6					8
					9		8	4
9			3		6			
1		7	2			9	5	

Puzzle 26 (Medium, difficulty rating 0.48)

		7		2	5			
					7	1		5
		9	8			2		
6	5	8		7				
9			3		6			2
			8			7	9	6
		5			1	9		
8		2	7					
			2	3		4		

Puzzle 27 (Easy, difficulty rating 0.42)

	9		5				8	6
		4	3	8				7
	5	7			6	9		
							5	4
		1		3		2		
3	6							
		8	7			6	9	
4				9	3	7		
2	7				1		4	

Puzzle 28 (Very hard, difficulty rating 0.79)

		5	4					
7					2			4
9		4	5	6	7			
				4		3		
	1	7	9		6	2	8	
		2		5				
			8	2	5	4		6
5			6					1
					4	5		

Puzzle 29 (Hard, difficulty rating 0.60)

8		5					3	
				5	9	7		
					4		1	5
			8	6	3			
	1	3	4		7	8	5	
		7	3	9				
3	9		5					
		2	9	7				
	4					5		2

Puzzle 30 (Medium, difficulty rating 0.57)

5				4		7		
		7		9				
1					6	5	2	4
	2			5		1	4	
3								5
	5	1		8			3	
2	8	4	6					3
			4			2		
		3		9				8

Puzzle 31 (Medium, difficulty rating 0.52)

8	4				6	2	7	
			7					1
		7			1			
	6	5	2		8			4
	1			7			8	
9			4		5	7	6	
			1			4		
4					3			
	2	8	9				5	3

Puzzle 32 (Very hard, difficulty rating 0.77)

	6					8		
9			2			7		
	1	7		9	8	3		2
			7	2	5			
3				8				9
			3	1	9			
5		1	8	3		9	4	
		9			2			3
		3					2	

Puzzle 33 (Medium, difficulty rating 0.49)

8						3		
	4	2	8	9	3			
	7		1		5			
2	1				4			3
	3			5			4	
6			2				7	9
			3		9		1	
			6	1	2	7	8	
		7						6

Puzzle 34 (Medium, difficulty rating 0.51)

		9	5					
6	3		7	8	2			
5	1		6					2
7			4					
	2		3		7		4	
					5			6
8					3		7	9
			8	5	6		3	4
					1	6		

Puzzle 35 (Medium, difficulty rating 0.57)

	3		7		1		9	
9				2				1
						4		
			4			1	7	5
1		7	2		5	8		9
4	8	5			9			
		9						
6				5				7
	2		9		4		3	

Puzzle 36 (Easy, difficulty rating 0.36)

							8	5
		8	6			2	4	
			2		8			7
	3		7			6	5	1
6				3				9
5	7	4			9		3	
1			3		2			
	6	5			7	3		
9	8							

Puzzle 37 (Easy, difficulty rating 0.41)

				7				2
4	7			8			6	
			5			9	7	
	1	6	8					5
		2	4	3	6	7		
7					5	8	2	
	8	7			2			
	6			5			1	9
2				6				

Puzzle 38 (Easy, difficulty rating 0.43)

6		5			2			
		4	9		7	1	2	
	7			6		8		3
				3	9			
	9						6	
		3	7					
2		8		7			3	
	3	7	1		4	6		
			5			2		4

Puzzle 39 (Medium, difficulty rating 0.51)

			3				4	9
	2	1	9		4			
		3	6				7	
	3	4			6	7		
	7			4			5	
		2	8			4	9	
	5				3	8		
			5			1	3	6
3	1				8			

Puzzle 40 (Easy, difficulty rating 0.44)

	6	4		9			7	
	8		1			6	3	
		1		7	6			4
	7			6				
		9				5		
				2			8	
3			5	1		7		
	5	6			8		1	
	4			3		8	2	

Puzzle 41 (Medium, difficulty rating 0.49)

	6			2		9		8
2		9	1	7		6		
			3					
		8				3	1	
7	2						8	9
	4	1				7		
					7			
		6		5	1	8		3
4		5		6			2	

Puzzle 42 (Easy, difficulty rating 0.41)

7	4		2					
8				1			2	5
	2			9	8	1		6
			7			3	1	
	1	8			9			
6		2	8	3			4	
1	8			2				9
					6		8	1

Puzzle 43 (Medium, difficulty rating 0.55)

4	5		3					
	9		5			4		
	8					5		3
2		9		3		8	1	
	7						2	
	1	8		2		3		7
6		1				5		
		5			4	8		
					2		3	9

Puzzle 44 (Easy, difficulty rating 0.31)

	7	9	8			6		
	5						8	
3	8	6		7				
4		3		2				1
		1		3		9		
5				6		8		2
				8		2	7	3
	1						4	
		2			4	1	9	

Puzzle 45 (Medium, difficulty rating 0.50)

					3			
			6		3		4	
	8		4	9	1			2
		7	2	5	6			
5		4				8		1
			8	1	4	2		
4		2		6	1		9	
	9		3		2			
		5						

Puzzle 46 (Easy, difficulty rating 0.41)

		7						
		6	1	4			9	7
			3		5	1		
	7	3	5	8		2		
	5			9			7	
		4		2	7	5	3	
		9	2		4			
3	4			5	8	9		
						8		

Puzzle 47 (Hard, difficulty rating 0.70)

				7	8			
5	7		9	3			4	
4		6				7		9
			3			5	2	
9								1
	2	5			6			
7		1				4		5
	6			4	3		1	7
		4	7					

Puzzle 48 (Medium, difficulty rating 0.59)

	4			5	9	8		2
	5		6	2				
				8				5
6				9			2	4
4				1				9
9	1			8				3
5			2					
				6	5		7	
3			1	8	4		5	

Puzzle 49

			7	9				
	2		8	4	3			
6	4	3	1					
		4				1	9	
5			4		8			6
	1	6				4		
					4	8	3	2
			9	8	1		7	
				5	2			

Puzzle 50

7	6		3			4	8	
		3			6	7		
				2	4		9	
						1		8
	9		8		2		6	
2		8						
	2		1	9				
		9	6			2		
	7	6			8		3	1

SOLUTIONS

SOLUTIONS TO THE SUDOKU PUZZLES	
Difficulty Level: Easy	75
Difficulty Level: Medium	80
Difficulty Level: Hard	85
Difficulty Level: Very Hard	90
Difficulty Level: Random	95

DIFFICULTY LEVEL - EASY

Puzzle 1 (Easy, difficulty rating 0.44)

5	3	2	1	4	6	7	9	8
4	7	6	9	8	2	5	1	3
8	9	1	7	3	5	2	6	4
9	4	5	8	6	3	1	7	2
3	1	8	2	7	9	4	5	6
2	6	7	4	5	1	8	3	9
6	8	3	5	2	7	9	4	1
7	2	9	6	1	4	3	8	5
1	5	4	3	9	8	6	2	7

Puzzle 2 (Easy, difficulty rating 0.35)

9	6	7	3	1	2	8	4	5
4	1	2	7	8	5	6	3	9
5	8	3	6	4	9	1	2	7
2	9	1	8	5	7	4	6	3
3	7	5	4	2	6	9	1	8
6	4	8	9	3	1	7	5	2
8	2	4	1	7	3	5	9	6
7	3	6	5	9	4	2	8	1
1	5	9	2	6	8	3	7	4

Puzzle 3 (Easy, difficulty rating 0.44)

9	7	6	2	5	1	4	3	8
2	1	3	6	8	4	7	5	9
4	5	8	7	9	3	2	6	1
6	9	4	1	3	7	5	8	2
1	8	7	4	2	5	6	9	3
3	2	5	8	6	9	1	7	4
7	6	1	9	4	8	3	2	5
8	3	2	5	1	6	9	4	7
5	4	9	3	7	2	8	1	6

Puzzle 4 (Easy, difficulty rating 0.38)

1	9	3	5	7	2	4	8	6
6	2	4	3	8	9	5	1	7
8	5	7	4	1	6	9	3	2
9	8	2	1	6	7	3	5	4
7	4	1	9	3	5	2	6	8
3	6	5	2	4	8	1	7	9
5	3	8	7	2	4	6	9	1
4	1	6	8	9	3	7	2	5
2	7	9	6	5	1	8	4	3

Puzzle 5 (Easy, difficulty rating 0.44)

8	1	9	6	2	7	5	3	4
2	4	3	5	1	9	8	7	6
7	6	5	8	4	3	2	1	9
3	7	6	4	8	2	1	9	5
5	2	8	9	7	1	6	4	3
1	9	4	3	5	6	7	2	8
4	3	7	2	6	8	9	5	1
9	8	1	7	3	5	4	6	2
6	5	2	1	9	4	3	8	7

Puzzle 6 (Easy, difficulty rating 0.40)

6	1	3	5	2	9	7	8	4
9	8	5	4	7	3	2	1	6
2	7	4	8	1	6	5	9	3
4	5	1	3	6	7	8	2	9
3	6	2	9	5	8	1	4	7
7	9	8	1	4	2	3	6	5
1	4	7	2	9	5	6	3	8
8	2	6	7	3	4	9	5	1
5	3	9	6	8	1	4	7	2

Puzzle 7 (Easy, difficulty rating 0.45)

5	9	3	7	1	8	6	4	2
8	4	2	3	6	9	7	1	5
1	6	7	5	4	2	9	3	8
7	1	8	6	5	3	2	9	4
2	3	4	8	9	7	5	6	1
6	5	9	1	2	4	8	7	3
4	7	5	2	3	6	1	8	9
3	8	1	9	7	5	4	2	6
9	2	6	4	8	1	3	5	7

Puzzle 8 (Easy, difficulty rating 0.36)

7	2	5	3	1	4	6	9	8
8	1	3	2	6	9	5	7	4
4	9	6	5	8	7	2	1	3
9	8	1	4	5	6	3	2	7
6	5	7	1	2	3	8	4	9
2	3	4	7	9	8	1	6	5
3	6	9	8	4	2	7	5	1
5	4	8	6	7	1	9	3	2
1	7	2	9	3	5	4	8	6

Puzzle 9 (Easy, difficulty rating 0.32)

1	5	8	7	3	2	4	6	9
7	2	6	4	9	8	3	1	5
9	4	3	5	1	6	7	8	2
6	3	4	8	7	5	9	2	1
8	1	7	2	6	9	5	4	3
2	9	5	3	4	1	8	7	6
5	6	2	9	8	7	1	3	4
4	8	1	6	5	3	2	9	7
3	7	9	1	2	4	6	5	8

Puzzle 10 (Easy, difficulty rating 0.38)

2	3	4	5	7	8	6	9	1
7	9	5	6	1	2	4	8	3
1	8	6	9	4	3	5	2	7
4	2	3	1	5	7	8	6	9
8	5	7	3	9	6	1	4	2
6	1	9	8	2	4	7	3	5
3	7	2	4	6	1	9	5	8
9	6	1	2	8	5	3	7	4
5	4	8	7	3	9	2	1	6

Puzzle 11 (Easy, difficulty rating 0.44)

5	1	2	7	9	4	8	6	3
4	9	6	8	3	1	2	5	7
3	8	7	2	6	5	4	1	9
1	7	4	6	5	2	3	9	8
2	5	3	4	8	9	6	7	1
9	6	8	3	1	7	5	2	4
7	3	5	9	2	8	1	4	6
8	2	9	1	4	6	7	3	5
6	4	1	5	7	3	9	8	2

Puzzle 12 (Easy, difficulty rating 0.35)

3	1	7	4	6	5	9	2	8
4	9	5	8	3	2	1	7	6
2	8	6	9	1	7	5	3	4
6	5	8	3	7	4	2	1	9
1	4	2	5	8	9	7	6	3
7	3	9	1	2	6	8	4	5
9	6	1	7	5	3	4	8	2
8	2	4	6	9	1	3	5	7
5	7	3	2	4	8	6	9	1

Puzzle 13 (Easy, difficulty rating 0.33)

4	1	7	3	8	9	2	5	6
6	8	3	1	5	2	4	9	7
2	9	5	6	4	7	3	1	8
3	2	9	5	7	4	6	8	1
7	4	8	9	1	6	5	3	2
1	5	6	2	3	8	7	4	9
8	6	2	4	9	5	1	7	3
5	7	1	8	6	3	9	2	4
9	3	4	7	2	1	8	6	5

Puzzle 14 (Easy, difficulty rating 0.42)

4	2	6	9	7	3	1	8	5
7	9	8	6	5	1	2	4	3
3	5	1	2	4	8	9	6	7
8	3	9	7	2	4	6	5	1
6	1	2	8	3	5	4	7	9
5	7	4	1	6	9	8	3	2
1	4	7	3	8	2	5	9	6
2	6	5	4	9	7	3	1	8
9	8	3	5	1	6	7	2	4

Puzzle 15 (Easy, difficulty rating 0.43)

9	2	8	7	5	1	4	6	3
3	1	6	9	2	4	5	7	8
4	7	5	8	6	3	1	9	2
8	6	4	3	9	5	7	2	1
5	3	2	1	4	7	6	8	9
7	9	1	2	8	6	3	4	5
1	8	7	6	3	2	9	5	4
6	5	9	4	1	8	2	3	7
2	4	3	5	7	9	8	1	6

Puzzle 16 (Easy, difficulty rating 0.37)

6	5	1	9	4	7	2	8	3
2	7	3	6	8	1	5	9	4
4	9	8	3	2	5	1	7	6
8	3	9	7	1	2	6	4	5
5	6	7	8	3	4	9	1	2
1	4	2	5	9	6	8	3	7
7	8	6	4	5	9	3	2	1
3	1	4	2	6	8	7	5	9
9	2	5	1	7	3	4	6	8

Puzzle 17 (Easy, difficulty rating 0.42)

7	9	2	4	3	8	1	6	5
5	1	8	6	2	7	4	9	3
3	4	6	5	9	1	2	8	7
8	2	3	9	1	5	7	4	6
1	5	4	8	7	6	3	2	9
6	7	9	3	4	2	5	1	8
4	6	7	2	5	9	8	3	1
9	3	1	7	8	4	6	5	2
2	8	5	1	6	3	9	7	4

Puzzle 18 (Easy, difficulty rating 0.30)

7	5	2	3	1	6	8	4	9
4	3	6	8	9	5	7	2	1
8	1	9	7	4	2	6	5	3
9	4	8	6	3	7	2	1	5
6	2	1	9	5	8	4	3	7
3	7	5	1	2	4	9	6	8
2	8	4	5	7	1	3	9	6
1	9	7	4	6	3	5	8	2
5	6	3	2	8	9	1	7	4

Puzzle 19 (Easy, difficulty rating 0.28)

4	5	3	1	7	2	9	8	6
1	9	2	8	4	6	3	5	7
8	7	6	5	9	3	4	1	2
6	8	9	4	1	7	5	2	3
7	3	4	2	5	9	1	6	8
2	1	5	3	6	8	7	9	4
3	6	1	7	2	5	8	4	9
9	4	8	6	3	1	2	7	5
5	2	7	9	8	4	6	3	1

Puzzle 20 (Easy, difficulty rating 0.26)

1	8	2	4	5	9	3	7	6
9	7	4	6	1	3	2	5	8
5	3	6	2	8	7	1	4	9
2	1	3	9	6	5	4	8	7
8	9	5	3	7	4	6	1	2
6	4	7	1	2	8	5	9	3
4	2	1	8	9	6	7	3	5
3	5	9	7	4	2	8	6	1
7	6	8	5	3	1	9	2	4

Puzzle 21 (Easy, difficulty rating 0.36)

8	6	1	2	5	7	9	4	3
2	9	4	6	1	3	5	7	8
7	5	3	9	8	4	6	1	2
6	1	7	5	4	2	3	8	9
9	4	2	8	3	6	7	5	1
5	3	8	7	9	1	4	2	6
4	8	6	3	2	5	1	9	7
3	2	5	1	7	9	8	6	4
1	7	9	4	6	8	2	3	5

Puzzle 22 (Easy, difficulty rating 0.40)

4	3	7	9	1	6	2	8	5
2	6	1	5	8	4	9	3	7
5	9	8	3	2	7	4	1	6
8	4	6	1	9	2	7	5	3
1	5	9	7	3	8	6	4	2
3	7	2	4	6	5	8	9	1
9	8	5	2	7	1	3	6	4
7	1	3	6	4	9	5	2	8
6	2	4	8	5	3	1	7	9

Puzzle 23 (Easy, difficulty rating 0.33)

8	6	3	4	2	5	9	7	1
5	7	9	8	3	1	2	4	6
1	2	4	9	7	6	5	3	8
6	3	1	5	8	7	4	2	9
9	8	7	6	4	2	3	1	5
4	5	2	3	1	9	8	6	7
7	9	5	2	6	3	1	8	4
3	1	8	7	9	4	6	5	2
2	4	6	1	5	8	7	9	3

Puzzle 24 (Easy, difficulty rating 0.35)

2	9	8	7	4	3	1	5	6
4	5	7	1	8	6	9	2	3
6	1	3	2	9	5	7	8	4
3	7	4	6	1	2	8	9	5
8	6	5	4	7	9	2	3	1
1	2	9	3	5	8	6	4	7
7	8	1	9	3	4	5	6	2
5	4	6	8	2	7	3	1	9
9	3	2	5	6	1	4	7	8

Puzzle 25 (Easy, difficulty rating 0.38)

6	5	3	7	4	1	9	2	8
1	4	9	2	8	3	5	6	7
7	8	2	5	6	9	1	3	4
2	9	5	6	1	4	8	7	3
8	3	1	9	7	2	4	5	6
4	6	7	3	5	8	2	9	1
5	7	8	1	9	6	3	4	2
9	2	4	8	3	7	6	1	5
3	1	6	4	2	5	7	8	9

Puzzle 26 (Easy, difficulty rating 0.44)

5	1	6	4	8	7	3	9	2
7	8	2	1	3	9	4	6	5
9	4	3	2	6	5	7	1	8
3	9	1	8	5	4	2	7	6
6	7	8	3	9	2	5	4	1
4	2	5	7	1	6	9	8	3
1	5	4	9	2	8	6	3	7
2	3	7	6	4	1	8	5	9
8	6	9	5	7	3	1	2	4

Puzzle 27 (Easy, difficulty rating 0.37)

3	7	2	6	4	8	9	1	5
6	8	1	5	2	9	7	3	4
5	9	4	7	3	1	6	8	2
4	5	8	1	6	7	2	9	3
1	3	9	8	5	2	4	7	6
7	2	6	3	9	4	1	5	8
2	1	5	9	8	6	3	4	7
8	6	7	4	1	3	5	2	9
9	4	3	2	7	5	8	6	1

Puzzle 28 (Easy, difficulty rating 0.37)

2	5	7	8	4	1	9	3	6
4	6	3	7	9	5	2	1	8
8	9	1	6	2	3	4	5	7
9	4	2	3	7	6	1	8	5
7	1	8	9	5	2	6	4	3
6	3	5	4	1	8	7	9	2
3	7	4	2	8	9	5	6	1
5	8	9	1	6	7	3	2	4
1	2	6	5	3	4	8	7	9

Puzzle 29 (Easy, difficulty rating 0.44)

5	3	8	9	2	7	1	4	6
2	4	9	6	1	3	8	5	7
6	1	7	8	4	5	9	2	3
3	8	1	5	9	6	4	7	2
9	7	5	4	3	2	6	8	1
4	6	2	7	8	1	3	9	5
1	9	3	2	7	4	5	6	8
7	5	4	1	6	8	2	3	9
8	2	6	3	5	9	7	1	4

Puzzle 30 (Easy, difficulty rating 0.39)

2	4	9	1	5	8	6	3	7
7	8	5	2	6	3	1	4	9
3	6	1	7	9	4	5	2	8
6	3	4	9	8	2	7	5	1
9	2	7	6	1	5	4	8	3
1	5	8	3	4	7	2	9	6
4	9	6	8	2	1	3	7	5
5	1	3	4	7	9	8	6	2
8	7	2	5	3	6	9	1	4

Puzzle 31 (Easy, difficulty rating 0.43)

8	7	9	1	2	4	6	5	3
2	1	3	7	5	6	4	8	9
6	4	5	9	3	8	1	7	2
9	6	1	8	7	3	2	4	5
5	2	4	6	1	9	7	3	8
7	3	8	2	4	5	9	1	6
3	5	2	4	6	1	8	9	7
4	8	7	3	9	2	5	6	1
1	9	6	5	8	7	3	2	4

Puzzle 32 (Easy, difficulty rating 0.42)

8	3	7	4	5	1	6	2	9
9	2	4	6	8	3	7	5	1
1	5	6	7	2	9	4	3	8
7	1	5	8	9	2	3	4	6
6	8	2	3	1	4	9	7	5
4	9	3	5	6	7	8	1	2
5	4	9	2	3	8	1	6	7
2	7	1	9	4	6	5	8	3
3	6	8	1	7	5	2	9	4

Puzzle 33 (Easy, difficulty rating 0.43)

9	1	7	5	4	3	8	6	2
4	5	8	2	6	1	3	9	7
2	3	6	8	9	7	4	5	1
8	7	9	1	2	5	6	4	3
3	6	1	9	7	4	5	2	8
5	2	4	3	8	6	1	7	9
6	4	2	7	1	8	9	3	5
7	8	3	6	5	9	2	1	4
1	9	5	4	3	2	7	8	6

Puzzle 34 (Easy, difficulty rating 0.42)

2	5	9	7	8	6	1	4	3
1	3	6	4	2	5	8	9	7
4	8	7	3	9	1	5	6	2
5	1	4	2	7	9	6	3	8
8	6	2	5	3	4	9	7	1
7	9	3	6	1	8	4	2	5
3	4	1	9	5	2	7	8	6
6	7	8	1	4	3	2	5	9
9	2	5	8	6	7	3	1	4

Puzzle 35 (Easy, difficulty rating 0.44)

6	2	5	3	4	9	7	8	1
9	3	1	8	5	7	2	4	6
7	8	4	1	6	2	9	5	3
4	9	8	2	3	5	6	1	7
3	6	7	9	1	4	8	2	5
1	5	2	7	8	6	4	3	9
2	1	6	5	7	8	3	9	4
8	7	3	4	9	1	5	6	2
5	4	9	6	2	3	1	7	8

Puzzle 36 (Easy, difficulty rating 0.36)

6	7	1	9	4	3	2	8	5
8	2	9	5	1	7	3	4	6
4	5	3	2	6	8	1	9	7
2	9	8	3	5	4	7	6	1
7	3	4	1	8	6	5	2	9
5	1	6	7	9	2	8	3	4
1	8	5	6	2	9	4	7	3
9	4	7	8	3	5	6	1	2
3	6	2	4	7	1	9	5	8

Puzzle 37 (Easy, difficulty rating 0.42)

2	7	3	8	5	1	9	6	4
1	6	4	9	7	2	8	5	3
5	9	8	6	3	4	7	2	1
4	5	1	7	9	8	6	3	2
3	2	9	5	4	6	1	8	7
6	8	7	1	2	3	4	9	5
9	1	2	4	8	5	3	7	6
8	4	5	3	6	7	2	1	9
7	3	6	2	1	9	5	4	8

Puzzle 38 (Easy, difficulty rating 0.44)

5	4	7	3	2	9	6	1	8
2	9	1	5	6	8	7	3	4
8	3	6	7	1	4	9	2	5
4	8	3	9	7	1	5	6	2
7	6	2	8	3	5	1	4	9
9	1	5	2	4	6	8	7	3
6	5	4	1	9	3	2	8	7
1	2	8	4	5	7	3	9	6
3	7	9	6	8	2	4	5	1

Puzzle 39 (Easy, difficulty rating 0.42)

3	9	2	4	7	5	8	1	6
1	7	6	8	2	3	5	9	4
8	5	4	9	1	6	2	7	3
6	1	3	7	5	2	9	4	8
2	8	7	6	9	4	1	3	5
5	4	9	1	3	8	7	6	2
9	2	8	3	6	1	4	5	7
4	6	1	5	8	7	3	2	9
7	3	5	2	4	9	6	8	1

Puzzle 40 (Easy, difficulty rating 0.28)

8	2	6	5	9	4	7	1	3
4	5	3	1	7	6	9	8	2
7	1	9	3	2	8	4	5	6
6	7	8	2	1	9	3	4	5
2	9	5	4	6	3	1	7	8
1	3	4	7	8	5	6	2	9
5	8	1	9	3	7	2	6	4
3	4	7	6	5	2	8	9	1
9	6	2	8	4	1	5	3	7

Puzzle 41 (Easy, difficulty rating 0.35)

3	4	2	8	9	1	7	6	5
1	7	5	2	3	6	8	4	9
9	6	8	4	7	5	3	1	2
2	8	6	3	5	4	1	9	7
7	1	3	6	8	9	2	5	4
5	9	4	1	2	7	6	3	8
8	5	1	9	6	2	4	7	3
4	3	7	5	1	8	9	2	6
6	2	9	7	4	3	5	8	1

Puzzle 42 (Easy, difficulty rating 0.42)

2	8	9	6	1	5	4	7	3
3	1	6	7	2	4	5	9	8
4	5	7	8	3	9	6	1	2
9	4	5	2	8	1	3	6	7
1	6	2	3	4	7	8	5	9
7	3	8	9	5	6	2	4	1
6	9	3	4	7	2	1	8	5
5	2	4	1	9	8	7	3	6
8	7	1	5	6	3	9	2	4

Puzzle 43 (Easy, difficulty rating 0.42)

6	2	9	8	5	1	4	7	3
3	1	4	7	6	2	9	5	8
7	5	8	4	3	9	6	1	2
2	8	3	5	9	7	1	6	4
5	6	7	1	4	8	2	3	9
4	9	1	3	2	6	5	8	7
9	7	5	2	1	3	8	4	6
1	3	2	6	8	4	7	9	5
8	4	6	9	7	5	3	2	1

Puzzle 44 (Easy, difficulty rating 0.32)

8	5	1	7	2	9	6	4	3
4	2	3	5	6	8	1	7	9
7	9	6	1	4	3	2	8	5
2	8	7	3	1	5	4	9	6
3	6	9	4	8	7	5	2	1
1	4	5	6	9	2	8	3	7
9	7	2	8	5	6	3	1	4
5	1	8	9	3	4	7	6	2
6	3	4	2	7	1	9	5	8

Puzzle 45 (Easy, difficulty rating 0.45)

9	1	2	6	5	4	8	3	7
7	5	8	1	3	9	2	6	4
6	4	3	2	7	8	1	5	9
4	3	5	8	1	6	9	7	2
1	9	7	4	2	3	6	8	5
8	2	6	5	9	7	3	4	1
3	8	1	7	4	2	5	9	6
2	6	4	9	8	5	7	1	3
5	7	9	3	6	1	4	2	8

Puzzle 46 (Easy, difficulty rating 0.42)

2	6	8	3	4	5	9	1	7
5	1	9	8	7	2	4	6	3
3	7	4	6	9	1	8	2	5
6	4	3	5	1	7	2	9	8
1	8	5	9	2	6	7	3	4
7	9	2	4	8	3	1	5	6
4	5	1	7	6	9	3	8	2
8	2	6	1	3	4	5	7	9
9	3	7	2	5	8	6	4	1

Puzzle 47 (Easy, difficulty rating 0.42)

7	8	6	5	9	4	1	3	2
3	5	4	6	2	1	7	8	9
9	2	1	7	8	3	5	6	4
2	3	7	4	1	5	8	9	6
5	6	9	2	7	8	3	4	1
1	4	8	9	3	6	2	7	5
8	7	2	1	6	9	4	5	3
6	1	5	3	4	7	9	2	8
4	9	3	8	5	2	6	1	7

Puzzle 48 (Easy, difficulty rating 0.35)

5	4	6	1	8	9	3	7	2
3	1	9	2	4	7	8	6	5
8	2	7	6	3	5	1	9	4
1	9	8	5	7	2	4	3	6
4	3	5	8	9	6	2	1	7
6	7	2	4	1	3	5	8	9
7	5	4	3	6	8	9	2	1
2	6	3	9	5	1	7	4	8
9	8	1	7	2	4	6	5	3

Puzzle 49 (Easy, difficulty rating 0.36)

3	9	2	4	7	5	8	1	6
1	7	6	8	2	3	5	9	4
8	5	4	9	1	6	2	7	3
6	1	3	7	5	2	9	4	8
2	8	7	6	9	4	1	3	5
5	4	9	1	3	8	7	6	2
9	2	8	3	6	1	4	5	7
4	6	1	5	8	7	3	2	9
7	3	5	2	4	9	6	8	1

Puzzle 50 (Easy, difficulty rating 0.39)

8	4	2	7	6	5	3	1	9
3	9	5	4	1	2	7	8	6
6	1	7	9	3	8	2	4	5
7	8	1	5	9	6	4	2	3
9	6	3	2	7	4	8	5	1
5	2	4	3	8	1	6	9	7
1	3	9	8	4	7	5	6	2
4	5	6	1	2	3	9	7	8
2	7	8	6	5	9	1	3	4

DIFFICULTY LEVEL: MEDIUM

Puzzle 1 (Medium, difficulty rating 0.56)

1	7	2	4	3	9	6	8	5
4	5	8	2	7	6	9	3	1
3	6	9	5	8	1	4	7	2
2	8	1	7	5	4	3	9	6
7	9	3	6	2	8	1	5	4
6	4	5	9	1	3	8	2	7
5	1	4	8	9	7	2	6	3
8	3	7	1	6	2	5	4	9
9	2	6	3	4	5	7	1	8

Puzzle 2 (Medium, difficulty rating 0.46)

8	7	6	2	5	4	1	9	3
9	2	5	3	6	1	8	4	7
3	4	1	9	7	8	6	5	2
2	5	3	6	4	9	7	1	8
6	8	4	5	1	7	3	2	9
1	9	7	8	3	2	5	6	4
4	1	9	7	8	5	2	3	6
7	6	2	1	9	3	4	8	5
5	3	8	4	2	6	9	7	1

Puzzle 3 (Medium, difficulty rating 0.50)

9	8	7	2	6	1	3	4	5
1	6	4	3	8	5	2	9	7
5	3	2	7	9	4	1	8	6
7	2	9	1	4	6	5	3	8
8	4	6	5	3	7	9	1	2
3	5	1	9	2	8	7	6	4
2	9	8	4	5	3	6	7	1
6	7	3	8	1	2	4	5	9
4	1	5	6	7	9	8	2	3

Puzzle 4 (Medium, difficulty rating 0.49)

9	1	2	4	3	6	5	8	7
5	3	8	7	9	1	6	4	2
4	6	7	5	2	8	3	1	9
8	7	5	1	6	9	2	3	4
3	4	6	2	8	7	9	5	1
2	9	1	3	5	4	8	7	6
7	8	3	6	4	2	1	9	5
6	5	4	9	1	3	7	2	8
1	2	9	8	7	5	4	6	3

Puzzle 5 (Medium, difficulty rating 0.52)

1	5	3	4	9	2	7	8	6
9	8	7	6	1	3	2	4	5
2	4	6	8	7	5	9	3	1
3	2	1	5	6	9	8	7	4
4	9	5	2	8	7	6	1	3
7	6	8	1	3	4	5	9	2
6	3	2	9	4	8	1	5	7
5	7	9	3	2	1	4	6	8
8	1	4	7	5	6	3	2	9

Puzzle 6 (Medium, difficulty rating 0.52)

6	8	5	7	4	2	1	9	3
1	7	9	3	5	6	8	4	2
2	3	4	9	8	1	6	7	5
7	6	1	5	2	9	3	8	4
9	2	8	4	1	3	5	6	7
4	5	3	8	6	7	2	1	9
3	1	6	2	9	4	7	5	8
8	9	2	1	7	5	4	3	6
5	4	7	6	3	8	9	2	1

Puzzle 7 (Medium, difficulty rating 0.59)

5	2	9	6	1	4	7	8	3
1	3	8	2	5	7	6	9	4
4	7	6	9	3	8	5	1	2
2	4	7	5	6	9	8	3	1
9	5	3	8	2	1	4	6	7
8	6	1	7	4	3	2	5	9
3	9	2	4	8	6	1	7	5
6	1	4	3	7	5	9	2	8
7	8	5	1	9	2	3	4	6

Puzzle 8 (Medium, difficulty rating 0.47)

5	4	8	2	3	1	9	7	6
7	1	9	5	4	6	3	8	2
3	2	6	9	8	7	5	1	4
1	5	3	7	6	2	8	4	9
8	9	7	3	5	4	6	2	1
4	6	2	1	9	8	7	3	5
6	3	1	8	2	5	4	9	7
9	7	4	6	1	3	2	5	8
2	8	5	4	7	9	1	6	3

Puzzle 9 (Medium, difficulty rating 0.55)

6	9	5	2	4	8	7	1	3
4	1	3	9	6	7	8	2	5
2	7	8	3	5	1	4	9	6
7	2	4	8	9	6	5	3	1
9	8	6	1	3	5	2	7	4
3	5	1	7	2	4	6	8	9
1	6	2	5	8	9	3	4	7
8	4	9	6	7	3	1	5	2
5	3	7	4	1	2	9	6	8

Puzzle 10 (Medium, difficulty rating 0.48)

1	4	9	7	3	2	6	5	8
6	8	3	5	1	9	4	7	2
7	2	5	4	6	8	3	1	9
2	5	7	3	8	4	9	6	1
3	9	8	6	5	1	2	4	7
4	6	1	2	9	7	8	3	5
9	3	6	8	7	5	1	2	4
5	1	4	9	2	6	7	8	3
8	7	2	1	4	3	5	9	6

Puzzle 11 (Medium, difficulty rating 0.53)

3	4	1	6	2	8	5	7	9
2	5	7	4	9	1	8	3	6
6	8	9	5	7	3	4	2	1
1	7	6	2	8	4	9	5	3
5	2	3	7	6	9	1	8	4
4	9	8	3	1	5	2	6	7
8	1	2	9	3	7	6	4	5
9	3	5	8	4	6	7	1	2
7	6	4	1	5	2	3	9	8

Puzzle 12 (Medium, difficulty rating 0.47)

6	9	8	4	5	3	2	7	1
5	4	3	2	1	7	9	6	8
2	7	1	9	8	6	3	5	4
9	5	2	1	6	8	7	4	3
4	1	7	3	2	9	5	8	6
3	8	6	5	7	4	1	2	9
7	2	4	6	9	1	8	3	5
1	3	5	8	4	2	6	9	7
8	6	9	7	3	5	4	1	2

Puzzle 13 (Medium, difficulty rating 0.53)

3	9	4	8	1	5	6	2	7
6	2	1	9	7	3	5	8	4
7	5	8	6	2	4	3	9	1
9	6	7	3	8	1	4	5	2
8	1	5	7	4	2	9	3	6
2	4	3	5	6	9	7	1	8
4	3	2	1	9	6	8	7	5
5	7	6	2	3	8	1	4	9
1	8	9	4	5	7	2	6	3

Puzzle 14 (Medium, difficulty rating 0.55)

9	3	7	2	8	5	4	1	6
5	8	4	3	6	1	2	9	7
1	6	2	9	4	7	8	3	5
3	9	1	8	7	6	5	4	2
8	2	5	4	1	9	6	7	3
4	7	6	5	2	3	9	8	1
6	1	9	7	5	8	3	2	4
7	4	8	6	3	2	1	5	9
2	5	3	1	9	4	7	6	8

Puzzle 15 (Medium, difficulty rating 0.46)

1	8	4	2	6	5	3	9	7
9	7	6	8	3	1	2	5	4
3	2	5	4	7	9	1	6	8
4	5	8	9	2	6	7	3	1
2	6	3	7	1	8	9	4	5
7	1	9	3	5	4	6	8	2
6	3	2	5	8	7	4	1	9
5	9	1	6	4	2	8	7	3
8	4	7	1	9	3	5	2	6

Puzzle 16 (Medium, difficulty rating 0.60)

6	4	8	7	2	3	9	5	1
9	7	3	1	6	5	8	4	2
2	5	1	4	9	8	7	3	6
8	3	4	6	1	7	2	9	5
5	1	6	9	8	2	3	7	4
7	2	9	5	3	4	6	1	8
4	8	2	3	7	1	5	6	9
1	6	7	2	5	9	4	8	3
3	9	5	8	4	6	1	2	7

Puzzle 17 (Medium, difficulty rating 0.53)

4	7	1	9	8	3	6	5	2
5	8	6	2	4	7	9	3	1
2	3	9	1	5	6	4	7	8
7	2	3	5	6	9	1	8	4
1	9	8	3	7	4	2	6	5
6	5	4	8	1	2	3	9	7
3	1	7	6	2	8	5	4	9
8	6	2	4	9	5	7	1	3
9	4	5	7	3	1	8	2	6

Puzzle 18 (Medium, difficulty rating 0.48)

7	8	3	1	5	9	6	4	2
6	2	1	3	4	8	5	9	7
9	5	4	6	2	7	1	3	8
8	1	5	4	7	6	3	2	9
2	9	7	8	3	1	4	6	5
3	4	6	5	9	2	7	8	1
4	3	8	2	1	5	9	7	6
5	6	9	7	8	3	2	1	4
1	7	2	9	6	4	8	5	3

Puzzle 19 (Medium, difficulty rating 0.47)

8	2	5	3	1	9	6	4	7
7	6	3	4	8	5	2	9	1
9	4	1	2	6	7	3	8	5
2	3	4	7	5	8	1	6	9
1	9	7	6	2	4	5	3	8
6	5	8	9	3	1	7	2	4
5	7	2	8	9	3	4	1	6
4	8	6	1	7	2	9	5	3
3	1	9	5	4	6	8	7	2

Puzzle 20 (Medium, difficulty rating 0.47)

6	1	2	5	8	9	3	7	4
4	7	8	6	3	1	5	2	9
9	3	5	4	7	2	8	6	1
5	4	3	7	1	6	2	9	8
2	6	9	8	5	3	4	1	7
7	8	1	2	9	4	6	5	3
1	9	6	3	2	8	7	4	5
3	2	7	1	4	5	9	8	6
8	5	4	9	6	7	1	3	2

Puzzle 21 (Medium, difficulty rating 0.49)

9	4	5	3	7	1	2	6	8
3	7	1	8	6	2	5	9	4
2	6	8	5	9	4	7	3	1
4	9	6	2	8	5	3	1	7
1	5	3	6	4	7	9	8	2
7	8	2	1	3	9	4	5	6
5	2	9	4	1	6	8	7	3
6	3	7	9	2	8	1	4	5
8	1	4	7	5	3	6	2	9

Puzzle 22 (Medium, difficulty rating 0.46)

8	6	4	7	1	3	2	5	9
3	7	9	8	2	5	1	4	6
1	5	2	9	4	6	3	8	7
2	1	8	5	9	4	6	7	3
5	3	7	6	8	1	4	9	2
4	9	6	3	7	2	5	1	8
9	2	5	1	6	8	7	3	4
6	8	1	4	3	7	9	2	5
7	4	3	2	5	9	8	6	1

Puzzle 23 (Medium, difficulty rating 0.46)

2	9	1	8	3	4	5	6	7
7	4	5	2	6	1	8	9	3
8	3	6	5	7	9	2	1	4
4	6	2	9	1	5	3	7	8
3	7	8	6	4	2	1	5	9
1	5	9	7	8	3	6	4	2
6	2	4	3	5	7	9	8	1
5	1	3	4	9	8	7	2	6
9	8	7	1	2	6	4	3	5

Puzzle 24 (Medium, difficulty rating 0.52)

4	5	3	2	8	9	7	1	6
8	2	1	3	6	7	5	9	4
6	9	7	4	1	5	8	2	3
1	3	5	9	7	8	4	6	2
9	7	6	1	2	4	3	5	8
2	4	8	6	5	3	1	7	9
3	1	4	7	9	2	6	8	5
7	8	9	5	3	6	2	4	1
5	6	2	8	4	1	9	3	7

Puzzle 25 (Medium, difficulty rating 0.54)

8	4	2	6	5	9	3	1	7
1	3	6	8	4	7	9	2	5
5	9	7	2	3	1	4	8	6
2	7	3	4	9	6	8	5	1
6	5	8	3	1	2	7	4	9
4	1	9	5	7	8	6	3	2
3	6	1	9	2	4	5	7	8
9	2	4	7	8	5	1	6	3
7	8	5	1	6	3	2	9	4

Puzzle 26 (Medium, difficulty rating 0.52)

4	5	8	1	2	6	7	9	3
9	1	3	4	8	7	2	5	6
7	6	2	3	9	5	4	1	8
5	3	9	6	4	8	1	2	7
6	2	1	5	7	9	3	8	4
8	4	7	2	3	1	5	6	9
1	9	4	8	5	3	6	7	2
3	8	6	7	1	2	9	4	5
2	7	5	9	6	4	8	3	1

Puzzle 27 (Medium, difficulty rating 0.56)

2	9	6	1	5	3	7	8	4
8	3	4	7	9	6	5	2	1
7	5	1	2	8	4	3	9	6
6	7	8	9	3	1	4	5	2
3	4	2	5	6	7	8	1	9
9	1	5	8	4	2	6	7	3
5	6	7	4	1	9	2	3	8
1	2	3	6	7	8	9	4	5
4	8	9	3	2	5	1	6	7

Puzzle 28 (Medium, difficulty rating 0.53)

5	7	1	6	9	3	2	4	8
9	3	6	2	8	4	1	7	5
8	4	2	5	1	7	6	3	9
7	8	9	3	2	5	4	6	1
2	6	5	1	4	9	7	8	3
3	1	4	7	6	8	5	9	2
1	5	3	9	7	6	8	2	4
4	9	7	8	5	2	3	1	6
6	2	8	4	3	1	9	5	7

Puzzle 29 (Medium, difficulty rating 0.48)

9	6	7	2	1	5	4	3	8
3	1	8	7	9	4	2	6	5
2	5	4	6	8	3	7	1	9
4	3	9	8	5	7	6	2	1
6	8	2	1	4	9	5	7	3
5	7	1	3	6	2	8	9	4
7	2	5	4	3	1	9	8	6
1	4	6	9	2	8	3	5	7
8	9	3	5	7	6	1	4	2

Puzzle 30 (Medium, difficulty rating 0.59)

4	6	5	9	2	1	7	8	3
8	3	2	7	6	5	9	4	1
1	7	9	3	8	4	5	2	6
9	2	1	6	4	3	8	5	7
3	5	7	2	1	8	4	6	9
6	4	8	5	7	9	3	1	2
5	9	6	4	3	2	1	7	8
7	8	4	1	9	6	2	3	5
2	1	3	8	5	7	6	9	4

Puzzle 31 (Medium, difficulty rating 0.59)

6	5	7	3	2	1	9	4	8
2	3	8	4	9	6	1	7	5
9	1	4	7	8	5	2	6	3
7	9	1	5	4	3	8	2	6
4	2	3	6	1	8	5	9	7
8	6	5	9	7	2	3	1	4
1	7	2	8	5	4	6	3	9
5	4	6	1	3	9	7	8	2
3	8	9	2	6	7	4	5	1

Puzzle 32 (Medium, difficulty rating 0.58)

7	8	5	4	9	6	1	2	3
6	3	4	2	1	5	9	8	7
1	9	2	7	8	3	5	6	4
2	4	7	1	3	9	6	5	8
3	5	9	8	6	2	7	4	1
8	1	6	5	7	4	3	9	2
5	7	8	6	2	1	4	3	9
9	6	1	3	4	8	2	7	5
4	2	3	9	5	7	8	1	6

Puzzle 33 (Medium, difficulty rating 0.46)

2	4	3	1	7	5	8	9	6
7	1	9	4	6	8	3	5	2
8	5	6	2	9	3	7	1	4
9	3	2	5	4	7	1	6	8
1	6	7	9	8	2	5	4	3
5	8	4	3	1	6	9	2	7
4	7	1	6	3	9	2	8	5
3	9	5	8	2	4	6	7	1
6	2	8	7	5	1	4	3	9

Puzzle 34 (Medium, difficulty rating 0.56)

5	6	8	9	7	3	4	2	1
2	3	9	1	6	4	8	5	7
1	7	4	8	5	2	6	3	9
4	1	7	5	8	9	3	6	2
3	5	6	2	4	7	1	9	8
8	9	2	3	1	6	5	7	4
7	8	3	4	2	5	9	1	6
9	2	1	6	3	8	7	4	5
6	4	5	7	9	1	2	8	3

Puzzle 35 (Medium, difficulty rating 0.54)

1	6	2	3	5	4	9	7	8
5	8	7	1	9	2	3	6	4
4	9	3	7	8	6	2	5	1
3	5	6	4	7	8	1	2	9
2	4	8	9	6	1	7	3	5
9	7	1	2	3	5	4	8	6
6	2	9	5	4	7	8	1	3
8	1	4	6	2	3	5	9	7
7	3	5	8	1	9	6	4	2

Puzzle 36 (Medium, difficulty rating 0.47)

1	7	6	8	3	9	5	4	2
8	5	3	2	1	4	9	6	7
9	2	4	5	7	6	3	1	8
7	4	9	6	5	2	8	3	1
2	6	1	3	9	8	7	5	4
3	8	5	7	4	1	2	9	6
6	1	2	9	8	3	4	7	5
5	9	8	4	6	7	1	2	3
4	3	7	1	2	5	6	8	9

Puzzle 37 (Medium, difficulty rating 0.59)

5	9	7	8	2	1	3	4	6
2	3	4	9	6	5	1	7	8
6	1	8	4	3	7	9	2	5
1	6	9	5	7	8	4	3	2
4	7	5	2	1	3	6	8	9
3	8	2	6	4	9	5	1	7
8	2	3	1	9	6	7	5	4
7	5	6	3	8	4	2	9	1
9	4	1	7	5	2	8	6	3

Puzzle 38 (Medium, difficulty rating 0.56)

3	6	5	1	8	9	7	4	2
9	7	1	6	2	4	8	3	5
2	4	8	5	7	3	6	1	9
4	5	3	9	6	7	1	2	8
7	8	9	2	4	1	3	5	6
6	1	2	8	3	5	4	9	7
5	9	7	4	1	8	2	6	3
8	2	4	3	5	6	9	7	1
1	3	6	7	9	2	5	8	4

Puzzle 39 (Medium, difficulty rating 0.51)

6	3	8	1	2	9	7	5	4
1	4	9	7	5	8	3	6	2
5	7	2	4	6	3	8	9	1
8	2	5	9	7	1	6	4	3
9	6	3	5	4	2	1	7	8
7	1	4	8	3	6	9	2	5
4	8	6	3	9	5	2	1	7
2	5	1	6	8	7	4	3	9
3	9	7	2	1	4	5	8	6

Puzzle 40 (Medium, difficulty rating 0.47)

4	9	7	1	5	8	3	2	6
3	8	5	2	4	6	9	1	7
2	6	1	3	7	9	5	8	4
7	5	2	8	1	4	6	9	3
9	3	6	7	2	5	1	4	8
1	4	8	6	9	3	2	7	5
8	1	4	5	6	2	7	3	9
6	7	9	4	3	1	8	5	2
5	2	3	9	8	7	4	6	1

Puzzle 41 (Medium, difficulty rating 0.60)

4	8	1	2	5	6	7	9	3
5	3	9	1	7	4	2	6	8
6	2	7	3	8	9	5	1	4
2	9	5	4	1	8	3	7	6
8	4	6	9	3	7	1	2	5
7	1	3	5	6	2	4	8	9
3	7	4	8	9	1	6	5	2
1	5	8	6	2	3	9	4	7
9	6	2	7	4	5	8	3	1

Puzzle 42 (Medium, difficulty rating 0.50)

9	7	3	8	1	2	6	5	4
1	2	5	3	6	4	9	8	7
6	4	8	7	5	9	1	3	2
5	3	7	1	9	8	2	4	6
4	9	6	5	2	3	8	7	1
2	8	1	6	4	7	5	9	3
8	6	4	2	7	5	3	1	9
7	5	2	9	3	1	4	6	8
3	1	9	4	8	6	7	2	5

Puzzle 43 (Medium, difficulty rating 0.53)

2	5	1	4	7	8	3	9	6
6	4	3	9	2	1	7	8	5
9	8	7	5	3	6	4	2	1
5	1	6	8	9	3	2	4	7
3	7	9	2	6	4	1	5	8
4	2	8	1	5	7	9	6	3
1	9	4	7	8	5	6	3	2
8	3	2	6	1	9	5	7	4
7	6	5	3	4	2	8	1	9

Puzzle 44 (Medium, difficulty rating 0.56)

8	6	4	5	7	3	9	1	2
3	1	9	6	2	8	5	7	4
7	2	5	9	4	1	3	8	6
5	7	6	3	9	4	8	2	1
9	4	1	8	5	2	7	6	3
2	8	3	7	1	6	4	5	9
6	9	7	2	3	5	1	4	8
1	3	8	4	6	7	2	9	5
4	5	2	1	8	9	6	3	7

Puzzle 45 (Medium, difficulty rating 0.57)

3	7	6	8	1	5	2	9	4
1	9	5	2	3	4	7	8	6
4	8	2	6	9	7	1	5	3
2	5	9	7	6	1	3	4	8
6	4	1	3	8	2	5	7	9
7	3	8	5	4	9	6	1	2
8	1	3	4	5	6	9	2	7
9	2	4	1	7	3	8	6	5
5	6	7	9	2	8	4	3	1

Puzzle 46 (Medium, difficulty rating 0.54)

1	3	7	5	8	2	9	6	4
8	2	5	4	9	6	1	7	3
6	4	9	7	3	1	8	5	2
5	7	2	1	4	9	3	8	6
4	1	6	3	5	8	7	2	9
3	9	8	2	6	7	4	1	5
7	5	1	9	2	3	6	4	8
2	8	3	6	7	4	5	9	1
9	6	4	8	1	5	2	3	7

Puzzle 47 (Medium, difficulty rating 0.60)

8	1	9	3	5	4	7	2	6
4	3	6	2	7	1	8	9	5
5	2	7	8	6	9	4	1	3
7	4	3	1	8	5	9	6	2
6	8	5	4	9	2	3	7	1
1	9	2	7	3	6	5	8	4
9	6	8	5	2	3	1	4	7
3	7	1	6	4	8	2	5	9
2	5	4	9	1	7	6	3	8

Puzzle 48 (Medium, difficulty rating 0.47)

6	2	1	9	8	3	5	4	7
4	7	9	6	2	5	8	3	1
3	5	8	1	4	7	9	2	6
8	9	4	7	1	6	3	5	2
7	1	5	8	3	2	4	6	9
2	6	3	4	5	9	1	7	8
5	8	6	2	9	4	7	1	3
1	4	7	3	6	8	2	9	5
9	3	2	5	7	1	6	8	4

Puzzle 49 (Medium, difficulty rating 0.54)

5	6	2	1	8	4	9	7	3
8	1	4	3	9	7	2	5	6
7	3	9	5	6	2	1	4	8
3	4	6	9	7	8	5	2	1
2	9	8	4	5	1	6	3	7
1	5	7	2	3	6	8	9	4
9	7	1	6	4	5	3	8	2
4	2	3	8	1	9	7	6	5
6	8	5	7	2	3	4	1	9

Puzzle 50 (Medium, difficulty rating 0.56)

5	4	2	8	1	3	6	7	9
8	7	9	2	6	4	1	5	3
1	6	3	9	5	7	4	2	8
7	3	1	5	9	6	2	8	4
4	5	8	7	3	2	9	1	6
2	9	6	1	4	8	5	3	7
6	1	4	3	7	5	8	9	2
3	8	5	4	2	9	7	6	1
9	2	7	6	8	1	3	4	5

DIFFICULTY LEVEL: HARD

Puzzle 1 (Hard, difficulty rating 0.66)

1	8	4	9	2	3	7	6	5
3	6	7	4	5	8	2	9	1
2	9	5	1	6	7	3	4	8
6	4	3	8	1	2	9	5	7
5	7	1	3	9	6	4	8	2
9	2	8	5	7	4	6	1	3
4	1	6	2	3	5	8	7	9
8	3	9	7	4	1	5	2	6
7	5	2	6	8	9	1	3	4

Puzzle 2 (Hard, difficulty rating 0.69)

3	6	8	1	7	9	2	5	4
9	4	2	8	6	5	1	7	3
1	7	5	2	4	3	6	8	9
6	1	9	7	5	4	3	2	8
7	5	4	3	8	2	9	1	6
2	8	3	9	1	6	5	4	7
5	9	1	4	3	8	7	6	2
8	2	6	5	9	7	4	3	1
4	3	7	6	2	1	8	9	5

Puzzle 3 (Hard, difficulty rating 0.65)

1	9	5	2	3	4	6	8	7
8	2	3	6	5	7	9	4	1
7	6	4	9	1	8	3	2	5
9	5	7	4	6	2	8	1	3
2	4	6	1	8	3	5	7	9
3	1	8	7	9	5	2	6	4
4	3	2	8	7	9	1	5	6
5	8	1	3	4	6	7	9	2
6	7	9	5	2	1	4	3	8

Puzzle 4 (Hard, difficulty rating 0.62)

1	7	3	5	4	9	2	6	8
2	4	5	8	6	3	9	7	1
6	8	9	7	2	1	4	3	5
8	6	1	9	7	5	3	4	2
3	9	2	1	8	4	6	5	7
7	5	4	6	3	2	1	8	9
5	2	6	4	9	8	7	1	3
9	1	7	3	5	6	8	2	4
4	3	8	2	1	7	5	9	6

Puzzle 5 (Hard, difficulty rating 0.71)

5	8	4	3	7	6	1	2	9
1	6	7	2	8	9	4	5	3
2	9	3	5	1	4	6	7	8
8	3	2	6	4	7	9	1	5
9	4	1	8	5	2	3	6	7
7	5	6	1	9	3	8	4	2
3	2	9	4	6	5	7	8	1
6	7	8	9	2	1	5	3	4
4	1	5	7	3	8	2	9	6

Puzzle 6 (Hard, difficulty rating 0.67)

7	2	8	6	1	4	9	5	3
4	3	1	9	5	2	8	7	6
5	9	6	7	3	8	4	2	1
1	6	3	2	4	5	7	9	8
9	4	5	8	7	3	1	6	2
2	8	7	1	9	6	3	4	5
8	5	4	3	6	9	2	1	7
6	7	2	4	8	1	5	3	9
3	1	9	5	2	7	6	8	4

Puzzle 7 (Hard, difficulty rating 0.66)

9	3	8	6	1	5	4	7	2
2	7	1	8	4	9	5	6	3
5	6	4	2	3	7	8	9	1
7	4	9	5	8	2	1	3	6
6	1	5	4	7	3	9	2	8
8	2	3	1	9	6	7	4	5
4	5	7	3	6	1	2	8	9
3	8	2	9	5	4	6	1	7
1	9	6	7	2	8	3	5	4

Puzzle 8 (Hard, difficulty rating 0.74)

2	1	9	8	7	5	6	3	4
3	6	4	1	9	2	8	7	5
7	8	5	6	3	4	9	2	1
6	2	3	5	4	9	1	8	7
8	4	1	2	6	7	5	9	3
9	5	7	3	8	1	4	6	2
5	7	8	4	2	6	3	1	9
1	9	6	7	5	3	2	4	8
4	3	2	9	1	8	7	5	6

Puzzle 9 (Hard, difficulty rating 0.61)

8	6	5	9	2	3	7	4	1
9	1	4	6	7	8	3	5	2
2	3	7	5	4	1	9	6	8
3	7	8	4	1	5	2	9	6
6	5	1	3	9	2	8	7	4
4	9	2	7	8	6	1	3	5
1	4	3	2	6	7	5	8	9
5	8	9	1	3	4	6	2	7
7	2	6	8	5	9	4	1	3

Puzzle 10 (Hard, difficulty rating 0.60)

3	9	2	4	7	5	8	1	6
1	7	6	8	2	3	5	9	4
8	5	4	9	1	6	2	7	3
6	1	3	7	5	2	9	4	8
2	8	7	6	9	4	1	3	5
5	4	9	1	3	8	7	6	2
9	2	8	3	6	1	4	5	7
4	6	1	5	8	7	3	2	9
7	3	5	2	4	9	6	8	1

Puzzle 11 (Hard, difficulty rating 0.74)

4	8	7	6	1	5	2	9	3
2	9	5	7	4	3	1	6	8
1	6	3	9	2	8	7	4	5
3	5	2	1	9	4	8	7	6
7	1	9	2	8	6	5	3	4
8	4	6	3	5	7	9	2	1
6	3	1	8	7	2	4	5	9
5	7	8	4	3	9	6	1	2
9	2	4	5	6	1	3	8	7

Puzzle 12 (Hard, difficulty rating 0.65)

4	1	7	8	3	5	6	9	2
9	5	3	2	6	4	7	8	1
6	2	8	9	1	7	3	4	5
2	3	4	6	7	8	5	1	9
5	9	6	1	4	3	8	2	7
8	7	1	5	2	9	4	3	6
3	4	9	7	5	2	1	6	8
7	6	2	3	8	1	9	5	4
1	8	5	4	9	6	2	7	3

Puzzle 13 (Hard, difficulty rating 0.63)

4	9	8	6	7	3	1	5	2
1	3	5	4	9	2	8	7	6
7	6	2	5	8	1	9	3	4
6	4	3	1	5	9	2	8	7
9	8	7	2	4	6	3	1	5
5	2	1	8	3	7	6	4	9
3	7	4	9	2	8	5	6	1
8	1	9	7	6	5	4	2	3
2	5	6	3	1	4	7	9	8

Puzzle 14 (Hard, difficulty rating 0.63)

2	1	8	6	5	4	7	3	9
3	5	7	9	8	1	6	4	2
9	6	4	3	2	7	5	8	1
5	9	2	4	3	6	1	7	8
4	3	1	8	7	2	9	6	5
8	7	6	5	1	9	4	2	3
7	4	3	2	9	5	8	1	6
1	8	9	7	6	3	2	5	4
6	2	5	1	4	8	3	9	7

Puzzle 15 (Hard, difficulty rating 0.70)

5	7	3	2	1	8	6	4	9
4	1	2	6	3	9	5	7	8
6	8	9	7	5	4	2	1	3
8	2	4	5	9	6	1	3	7
7	9	5	3	8	1	4	2	6
3	6	1	4	7	2	9	8	5
1	5	7	9	4	3	8	6	2
9	4	6	8	2	7	3	5	1
2	3	8	1	6	5	7	9	4

Puzzle 16 (Hard, difficulty rating 0.70)

2	1	4	7	9	5	6	3	8
7	6	3	2	4	8	1	5	9
8	9	5	3	6	1	7	4	2
4	7	9	6	5	2	8	1	3
1	2	8	4	3	7	9	6	5
3	5	6	1	8	9	2	7	4
9	8	1	5	7	3	4	2	6
6	3	2	8	1	4	5	9	7
5	4	7	9	2	6	3	8	1

Puzzle 17 (Hard, difficulty rating 0.62)

9	6	5	1	2	4	7	3	8
3	4	8	9	5	7	1	6	2
2	7	1	6	8	3	4	9	5
4	8	6	3	7	1	2	5	9
5	9	7	2	4	8	3	1	6
1	3	2	5	6	9	8	7	4
6	2	4	7	1	5	9	8	3
7	5	9	8	3	2	6	4	1
8	1	3	4	9	6	5	2	7

Puzzle 18 (Hard, difficulty rating 0.67)

9	3	8	4	2	6	1	5	7
4	7	2	1	3	5	9	8	6
6	5	1	9	8	7	3	4	2
3	8	6	7	4	9	5	2	1
1	9	5	2	6	8	7	3	4
7	2	4	3	5	1	6	9	8
8	6	9	5	7	2	4	1	3
2	1	3	6	9	4	8	7	5
5	4	7	8	1	3	2	6	9

Puzzle 19 (Hard, difficulty rating 0.64)

1	8	7	4	2	9	5	6	3
3	6	4	8	5	7	1	2	9
5	9	2	6	3	1	8	4	7
6	7	5	2	8	4	3	9	1
9	4	3	5	1	6	7	8	2
8	2	1	9	7	3	4	5	6
4	3	9	1	6	8	2	7	5
2	1	6	7	4	5	9	3	8
7	5	8	3	9	2	6	1	4

Puzzle 20 (Hard, difficulty rating 0.64)

1	9	2	6	8	5	3	4	7
8	5	3	7	9	4	2	1	6
7	6	4	3	2	1	9	5	8
9	4	1	5	7	3	8	6	2
6	3	7	2	4	8	1	9	5
2	8	5	1	6	9	4	7	3
4	2	8	9	5	7	6	3	1
3	7	6	4	1	2	5	8	9
5	1	9	8	3	6	7	2	4

Puzzle 21 (Hard, difficulty rating 0.70)

7	4	1	6	8	3	9	5	2
6	5	8	2	9	4	3	1	7
2	3	9	7	5	1	8	6	4
4	1	6	9	3	5	7	2	8
5	2	3	8	4	7	1	9	6
8	9	7	1	6	2	4	3	5
1	6	2	3	7	8	5	4	9
3	8	5	4	2	9	6	7	1
9	7	4	5	1	6	2	8	3

Puzzle 22 (Hard, difficulty rating 0.64)

9	4	1	3	2	7	6	5	8
2	8	3	6	5	1	9	7	4
5	6	7	8	4	9	3	1	2
6	7	9	5	8	4	1	2	3
3	5	8	9	1	2	7	4	6
4	1	2	7	6	3	5	8	9
8	9	5	2	7	6	4	3	1
1	2	6	4	3	5	8	9	7
7	3	4	1	9	8	2	6	5

Puzzle 23 (Hard, difficulty rating 0.61)

4	5	8	2	3	9	1	6	7
6	2	7	4	1	8	5	9	3
9	1	3	5	6	7	4	2	8
3	6	5	1	9	4	8	7	2
8	9	4	7	2	3	6	5	1
1	7	2	8	5	6	3	4	9
7	8	6	9	4	1	2	3	5
5	3	9	6	8	2	7	1	4
2	4	1	3	7	5	9	8	6

Puzzle 24 (Hard, difficulty rating 0.60)

1	9	8	7	4	6	3	2	5
4	7	5	2	3	8	9	6	1
2	3	6	5	1	9	4	7	8
3	4	7	8	5	1	2	9	6
6	8	2	4	9	3	5	1	7
9	5	1	6	7	2	8	3	4
7	2	3	1	8	5	6	4	9
8	1	9	3	6	4	7	5	2
5	6	4	9	2	7	1	8	3

Puzzle 25 (Hard, difficulty rating 0.60)

6	2	8	7	3	5	4	1	9
3	5	9	1	8	4	2	6	7
1	4	7	9	6	2	3	5	8
9	7	5	2	4	6	8	3	1
4	8	1	3	5	9	7	2	6
2	6	3	8	7	1	9	4	5
8	1	4	5	9	3	6	7	2
7	3	2	6	1	8	5	9	4
5	9	6	4	2	7	1	8	3

Puzzle 26 (Hard, difficulty rating 0.71)

4	7	2	9	3	6	5	1	8
6	3	1	4	8	5	9	7	2
9	5	8	1	7	2	3	4	6
2	6	4	5	9	1	7	8	3
5	8	7	3	2	4	1	6	9
3	1	9	8	6	7	4	2	5
8	4	5	6	1	3	2	9	7
7	9	3	2	4	8	6	5	1
1	2	6	7	5	9	8	3	4

Puzzle 27 (Hard, difficulty rating 0.64)

1	8	4	3	6	9	7	2	5
3	5	2	8	4	7	9	6	1
6	9	7	5	2	1	8	4	3
2	1	5	4	8	3	6	7	9
9	4	6	2	7	5	3	1	8
7	3	8	1	9	6	2	5	4
8	6	1	9	5	2	4	3	7
5	2	9	7	3	4	1	8	6
4	7	3	6	1	8	5	9	2

Puzzle 28 (Hard, difficulty rating 0.63)

5	6	7	3	4	9	8	2	1
8	4	3	1	5	2	6	9	7
9	2	1	6	8	7	3	4	5
7	9	5	8	3	4	2	1	6
4	3	6	2	7	1	5	8	9
1	8	2	5	9	6	7	3	4
3	7	8	9	1	5	4	6	2
6	5	9	4	2	8	1	7	3
2	1	4	7	6	3	9	5	8

Puzzle 29 (Hard, difficulty rating 0.60)

4	5	2	3	1	8	6	9	7
3	1	9	7	2	6	8	4	5
6	8	7	4	9	5	3	2	1
1	4	5	9	3	7	2	6	8
9	2	6	5	8	1	7	3	4
7	3	8	2	6	4	1	5	9
5	6	1	8	4	3	9	7	2
2	7	3	1	5	9	4	8	6
8	9	4	6	7	2	5	1	3

Puzzle 30 (Hard, difficulty rating 0.67)

4	8	5	9	3	2	7	6	1
7	2	9	4	1	6	3	5	8
3	6	1	8	7	5	4	9	2
2	4	8	1	9	7	6	3	5
9	3	6	5	8	4	2	1	7
1	5	7	2	6	3	9	8	4
5	9	4	3	2	1	8	7	6
8	7	2	6	5	9	1	4	3
6	1	3	7	4	8	5	2	9

Puzzle 31 (Hard, difficulty rating 0.70)

4	6	7	5	1	8	2	9	3
5	3	2	6	7	9	8	1	4
9	8	1	2	4	3	7	5	6
6	1	4	7	3	2	9	8	5
7	9	8	1	5	6	4	3	2
2	5	3	9	8	4	1	6	7
3	7	9	4	6	1	5	2	8
8	2	5	3	9	7	6	4	1
1	4	6	8	2	5	3	7	9

Puzzle 32 (Hard, difficulty rating 0.60)

2	1	4	6	7	9	5	8	3
8	3	9	4	5	1	7	2	6
5	6	7	8	2	3	1	9	4
7	9	3	1	6	5	8	4	2
6	8	5	2	3	4	9	7	1
4	2	1	9	8	7	3	6	5
3	7	6	5	9	2	4	1	8
1	5	2	7	4	8	6	3	9
9	4	8	3	1	6	2	5	7

Puzzle 33 (Hard, difficulty rating 0.65)

8	4	1	3	5	6	2	7	9
6	5	2	7	9	4	8	3	1
3	9	7	8	2	1	5	4	6
7	6	5	2	3	8	9	1	4
2	1	4	6	7	9	3	8	5
9	8	3	4	1	5	7	6	2
5	3	6	1	8	2	4	9	7
4	7	9	5	6	3	1	2	8
1	2	8	9	4	7	6	5	3

Puzzle 34 (Hard, difficulty rating 0.61)

6	5	8	9	3	1	2	7	4
3	4	9	7	2	6	5	1	8
2	7	1	8	5	4	3	9	6
8	1	3	2	6	9	4	5	7
5	2	6	1	4	7	9	8	3
4	9	7	5	8	3	6	2	1
9	3	2	6	1	8	7	4	5
1	6	5	4	7	2	8	3	9
7	8	4	3	9	5	1	6	2

Puzzle 35 (Hard, difficulty rating 0.70)

1	2	5	6	7	4	8	3	9
4	6	3	9	8	2	1	5	7
9	7	8	5	3	1	2	6	4
7	9	2	8	4	3	5	1	6
6	3	1	7	2	5	4	9	8
8	5	4	1	6	9	7	2	3
3	4	9	2	1	8	6	7	5
2	8	6	3	5	7	9	4	1
5	1	7	4	9	6	3	8	2

Puzzle 36 (Hard, difficulty rating 0.62)

7	6	9	5	8	1	3	4	2
8	2	4	3	6	7	9	1	5
1	3	5	9	2	4	8	7	6
5	8	6	1	7	3	2	9	4
4	1	2	6	5	9	7	3	8
9	7	3	2	4	8	6	5	1
3	5	8	7	1	6	4	2	9
6	9	1	4	3	2	5	8	7
2	4	7	8	9	5	1	6	3

Puzzle 37 (Hard, difficulty rating 0.61)

7	1	4	3	2	8	9	6	5
8	5	2	6	1	9	4	3	7
3	9	6	5	7	4	8	2	1
5	6	1	2	8	3	7	9	4
9	3	8	7	4	5	6	1	2
2	4	7	1	9	6	3	5	8
6	7	3	4	5	2	1	8	9
1	2	9	8	3	7	5	4	6
4	8	5	9	6	1	2	7	3

Puzzle 38 (Hard, difficulty rating 0.64)

9	3	8	4	2	6	1	5	7
4	7	2	1	3	5	9	8	6
6	5	1	9	8	7	3	4	2
3	8	6	7	4	9	5	2	1
1	9	5	2	6	8	7	3	4
7	2	4	3	5	1	6	9	8
8	6	9	5	7	2	4	1	3
2	1	3	6	9	4	8	7	5
5	4	7	8	1	3	2	6	9

Puzzle 39 (Hard, difficulty rating 0.60)

1	2	3	6	8	5	4	9	7
8	9	5	4	2	7	6	3	1
7	6	4	1	9	3	5	8	2
9	5	2	8	4	1	7	6	3
4	8	1	7	3	6	2	5	9
3	7	6	9	5	2	1	4	8
5	1	7	3	6	8	9	2	4
2	4	8	5	7	9	3	1	6
6	3	9	2	1	4	8	7	5

Puzzle 40 (Hard, difficulty rating 0.66)

6	7	8	2	1	4	5	3	9
3	5	4	9	6	8	7	2	1
2	1	9	7	3	5	8	4	6
9	2	1	6	7	3	4	5	8
7	8	5	4	2	9	6	1	3
4	3	6	8	5	1	9	7	2
1	4	3	5	8	6	2	9	7
8	9	7	3	4	2	1	6	5
5	6	2	1	9	7	3	8	4

Puzzle 41 (Hard, difficulty rating 0.61)

2	8	6	5	1	9	4	3	7
5	1	3	4	2	7	9	6	8
4	9	7	6	8	3	5	1	2
6	7	8	2	5	4	3	9	1
3	5	9	1	7	6	8	2	4
1	4	2	9	3	8	6	7	5
9	6	5	7	4	2	1	8	3
7	3	1	8	6	5	2	4	9
8	2	4	3	9	1	7	5	6

Puzzle 42 (Hard, difficulty rating 0.70)

7	4	6	2	5	1	9	8	3
5	3	9	8	7	4	1	2	6
8	1	2	9	6	3	7	5	4
1	2	5	6	3	7	8	4	9
3	9	7	4	2	8	5	6	1
6	8	4	1	9	5	3	7	2
4	5	1	3	8	2	6	9	7
9	7	3	5	4	6	2	1	8
2	6	8	7	1	9	4	3	5

Puzzle 43 (Hard, difficulty rating 0.65)

3	7	2	9	4	6	5	8	1
8	4	9	1	5	7	3	6	2
5	1	6	8	2	3	4	7	9
9	3	8	6	1	5	7	2	4
1	2	7	3	8	4	9	5	6
4	6	5	2	7	9	8	1	3
2	9	1	7	3	8	6	4	5
6	8	4	5	9	2	1	3	7
7	5	3	4	6	1	2	9	8

Puzzle 44 (Hard, difficulty rating 0.68)

2	4	8	6	1	9	7	5	3
1	3	6	5	8	7	2	9	4
5	7	9	4	2	3	6	1	8
7	8	2	1	9	4	3	6	5
4	1	5	3	7	6	8	2	9
6	9	3	2	5	8	4	7	1
9	6	7	8	3	5	1	4	2
3	2	4	9	6	1	5	8	7
8	5	1	7	4	2	9	3	6

Puzzle 45 (Hard, difficulty rating 0.75)

7	3	9	2	6	1	5	8	4
2	1	8	5	3	4	9	6	7
4	6	5	9	8	7	3	2	1
3	5	1	7	2	8	6	4	9
8	2	4	3	9	6	7	1	5
6	9	7	1	4	5	2	3	8
1	7	2	4	5	3	8	9	6
5	8	3	6	1	9	4	7	2
9	4	6	8	7	2	1	5	3

Puzzle 46 (Hard, difficulty rating 0.63)

4	6	5	9	2	1	7	8	3
8	3	2	7	6	5	9	4	1
1	7	9	3	8	4	5	2	6
9	2	1	6	4	3	8	5	7
3	5	7	2	1	8	4	6	9
6	4	8	5	7	9	3	1	2
5	9	6	4	3	2	1	7	8
7	8	4	1	9	6	2	3	5
2	1	3	8	5	7	6	9	4

Puzzle 47 (Hard, difficulty rating 0.60)

9	7	5	2	3	1	6	4	8
4	1	3	9	6	8	7	5	2
2	8	6	7	5	4	9	3	1
7	5	1	6	8	2	4	9	3
8	4	9	3	1	5	2	7	6
6	3	2	4	7	9	1	8	5
5	2	7	8	9	6	3	1	4
1	9	4	5	2	3	8	6	7
3	6	8	1	4	7	5	2	9

Puzzle 48 (Hard, difficulty rating 0.63)

6	8	5	2	4	7	1	3	9
3	2	7	1	5	9	6	8	4
4	1	9	6	8	3	2	7	5
9	7	6	3	2	5	8	4	1
2	5	8	7	1	4	9	6	3
1	3	4	8	9	6	5	2	7
5	9	3	4	6	8	7	1	2
7	6	2	9	3	1	4	5	8
8	4	1	5	7	2	3	9	6

Puzzle 49 (Hard, difficulty rating 0.66)

4	7	1	2	3	9	8	6	5
8	5	9	6	7	4	2	3	1
3	2	6	8	5	1	4	9	7
5	1	7	4	8	3	9	2	6
2	6	8	9	1	7	3	5	4
9	4	3	5	2	6	1	7	8
1	3	4	7	6	2	5	8	9
6	9	5	3	4	8	7	1	2
7	8	2	1	9	5	6	4	3

Puzzle 50 (Hard, difficulty rating 0.63)

6	7	1	9	4	3	2	8	5
8	2	9	5	1	7	3	4	6
4	5	3	2	6	8	1	9	7
2	9	8	3	5	4	7	6	1
7	3	4	1	8	6	5	2	9
5	1	6	7	9	2	8	3	4
1	8	5	6	2	9	4	7	3
9	4	7	8	3	5	6	1	2
3	6	2	4	7	1	9	5	8

DIFFICULTY LEVEL: VERY HARD

Puzzle 1 (Very hard, difficulty rating 0.76)

7	9	5	1	8	4	3	2	6
3	1	6	5	9	2	8	7	4
8	4	2	6	3	7	1	5	9
6	3	4	8	2	1	7	9	5
9	5	1	3	7	6	2	4	8
2	7	8	9	4	5	6	3	1
4	6	3	2	1	9	5	8	7
5	2	7	4	6	8	9	1	3
1	8	9	7	5	3	4	6	2

Puzzle 2 (Very hard, difficulty rating 0.80)

4	6	1	8	2	7	9	5	3
9	8	2	4	5	3	7	1	6
3	7	5	6	1	9	4	2	8
8	9	3	2	7	1	5	6	4
6	1	7	3	4	5	8	9	2
2	5	4	9	6	8	3	7	1
5	3	6	7	8	2	1	4	9
1	4	9	5	3	6	2	8	7
7	2	8	1	9	4	6	3	5

Puzzle 3 (Very hard, difficulty rating 0.78)

2	5	6	9	7	4	8	3	1
8	3	9	1	2	5	6	4	7
4	1	7	6	3	8	5	2	9
6	7	5	2	4	9	3	1	8
9	8	4	3	6	1	2	7	5
1	2	3	5	8	7	9	6	4
7	6	8	4	9	3	1	5	2
3	9	1	7	5	2	4	8	6
5	4	2	8	1	6	7	9	3

Puzzle 4 (Very hard, difficulty rating 0.78)

7	2	6	4	1	3	9	8	5
4	8	9	2	6	5	1	3	7
5	3	1	8	7	9	2	6	4
9	5	2	1	4	8	3	7	6
3	6	7	5	9	2	4	1	8
8	1	4	7	3	6	5	9	2
6	4	5	9	8	1	7	2	3
2	9	8	3	5	7	6	4	1
1	7	3	6	2	4	8	5	9

Puzzle 5 (Very hard, difficulty rating 0.77)

9	3	4	6	1	5	2	8	7
7	5	2	3	4	8	6	1	9
8	1	6	9	7	2	5	4	3
1	6	7	4	5	9	3	2	8
5	2	3	7	8	1	9	6	4
4	8	9	2	6	3	7	5	1
2	9	5	8	3	4	1	7	6
6	4	1	5	9	7	8	3	2
3	7	8	1	2	6	4	9	5

Puzzle 6 (Very hard, difficulty rating 0.85)

8	5	7	9	2	3	6	1	4
4	3	9	6	1	7	2	5	8
6	2	1	8	4	5	3	7	9
2	1	8	7	3	9	5	4	6
3	6	4	2	5	1	9	8	7
7	9	5	4	8	6	1	2	3
9	7	2	1	6	4	8	3	5
1	4	3	5	9	8	7	6	2
5	8	6	3	7	2	4	9	1

Puzzle 7 (Very hard, difficulty rating 0.77)

9	1	6	8	7	3	5	4	2
7	3	8	4	2	5	6	1	9
5	4	2	6	9	1	3	8	7
6	7	9	1	5	4	2	3	8
4	2	3	7	6	8	9	5	1
1	8	5	9	3	2	7	6	4
3	9	1	5	8	7	4	2	6
8	5	7	2	4	6	1	9	3
2	6	4	3	1	9	8	7	5

Puzzle 8 (Very hard, difficulty rating 0.79)

9	3	2	1	6	5	4	8	7
7	1	4	8	3	9	2	5	6
5	8	6	7	2	4	9	3	1
1	2	7	6	4	8	5	9	3
3	5	9	2	7	1	6	4	8
6	4	8	9	5	3	7	1	2
2	9	1	4	8	7	3	6	5
8	7	3	5	9	6	1	2	4
4	6	5	3	1	2	8	7	9

Puzzle 9 (Very hard, difficulty rating 0.80)

6	2	5	7	4	1	8	3	9
8	4	9	2	3	6	1	7	5
1	3	7	8	5	9	4	6	2
2	8	6	3	1	5	9	4	7
9	5	1	4	7	8	3	2	6
3	7	4	9	6	2	5	8	1
4	6	2	1	9	3	7	5	8
7	9	8	5	2	4	6	1	3
5	1	3	6	8	7	2	9	4

Puzzle 10 (Very hard, difficulty rating 0.75)

3	2	4	1	6	9	7	8	5
7	5	1	3	2	8	4	9	6
6	8	9	7	4	5	2	3	1
9	4	2	8	5	7	6	1	3
5	3	7	6	1	4	8	2	9
1	6	8	9	3	2	5	7	4
4	9	6	2	8	3	1	5	7
8	7	5	4	9	1	3	6	2
2	1	3	5	7	6	9	4	8

Puzzle 11 (Very hard, difficulty rating 0.83)

5	4	1	8	6	3	9	2	7
9	2	3	5	7	4	6	8	1
8	7	6	9	1	2	5	3	4
1	3	7	2	5	8	4	6	9
2	5	8	4	9	6	7	1	3
4	6	9	7	3	1	2	5	8
3	1	5	6	4	9	8	7	2
7	8	4	1	2	5	3	9	6
6	9	2	3	8	7	1	4	5

Puzzle 12 (Very hard, difficulty rating 0.84)

6	9	8	1	5	2	3	4	7
4	7	1	9	3	8	6	2	5
5	3	2	6	4	7	8	1	9
7	4	9	3	8	5	2	6	1
3	1	6	2	7	9	5	8	4
8	2	5	4	1	6	7	9	3
2	5	7	8	9	1	4	3	6
1	6	3	5	2	4	9	7	8
9	8	4	7	6	3	1	5	2

Puzzle 13 (Very hard, difficulty rating 0.90)

3	9	5	4	7	6	1	8	2
6	2	7	5	8	1	4	9	3
1	8	4	9	3	2	7	5	6
8	5	1	6	2	9	3	4	7
4	7	9	8	1	3	6	2	5
2	3	6	7	5	4	8	1	9
5	6	3	1	9	8	2	7	4
7	4	8	2	6	5	9	3	1
9	1	2	3	4	7	5	6	8

Puzzle 14 (Very hard, difficulty rating 0.96)

5	7	4	2	1	9	8	3	6
1	3	6	8	4	5	9	2	7
8	2	9	7	3	6	1	4	5
4	8	3	9	2	7	5	6	1
2	6	7	1	5	3	4	9	8
9	1	5	4	6	8	3	7	2
3	9	1	5	7	2	6	8	4
7	5	8	6	9	4	2	1	3
6	4	2	3	8	1	7	5	9

Puzzle 15 (Very hard, difficulty rating 0.76)

1	7	6	5	2	9	3	8	4
9	2	5	4	8	3	7	1	6
4	8	3	6	7	1	2	5	9
3	9	2	8	1	4	5	6	7
5	4	7	3	9	6	8	2	1
6	1	8	7	5	2	4	9	3
2	3	9	1	4	5	6	7	8
8	6	1	2	3	7	9	4	5
7	5	4	9	6	8	1	3	2

Puzzle 16 (Very hard, difficulty rating 0.81)

9	5	8	6	7	4	2	1	3
4	1	7	3	5	2	6	8	9
3	2	6	8	9	1	4	5	7
2	8	1	4	6	7	3	9	5
5	7	4	9	2	3	1	6	8
6	9	3	1	8	5	7	2	4
1	6	5	7	3	9	8	4	2
8	3	2	5	4	6	9	7	1
7	4	9	2	1	8	5	3	6

Puzzle 17 (Very hard, difficulty rating 0.91)

4	9	6	5	3	2	8	7	1
2	5	1	8	6	7	3	4	9
8	7	3	1	9	4	6	5	2
9	1	2	6	4	3	5	8	7
5	6	4	7	8	1	9	2	3
7	3	8	2	5	9	4	1	6
6	8	7	9	1	5	2	3	4
3	2	9	4	7	8	1	6	5
1	4	5	3	2	6	7	9	8

Puzzle 18 (Very hard, difficulty rating 0.81)

9	2	8	6	3	4	1	5	7
7	5	3	9	2	1	8	6	4
4	1	6	5	7	8	9	2	3
3	4	5	7	6	9	2	1	8
1	8	7	2	4	5	6	3	9
2	6	9	8	1	3	4	7	5
5	9	2	3	8	6	7	4	1
6	3	4	1	9	7	5	8	2
8	7	1	4	5	2	3	9	6

Puzzle 19 (Very hard, difficulty rating 0.83)

6	5	3	1	8	4	9	2	7
8	9	1	2	7	3	4	6	5
4	2	7	6	5	9	8	1	3
3	6	8	7	1	5	2	4	9
7	1	5	9	4	2	6	3	8
2	4	9	3	6	8	5	7	1
1	3	4	5	9	6	7	8	2
9	8	2	4	3	7	1	5	6
5	7	6	8	2	1	3	9	4

Puzzle 20 (Very hard, difficulty rating 0.98)

4	5	9	3	7	2	1	8	6
7	3	1	8	6	9	2	5	4
6	8	2	4	1	5	3	9	7
5	6	4	2	9	3	8	7	1
9	1	3	7	4	8	5	6	2
8	2	7	1	5	6	9	4	3
3	4	5	6	8	1	7	2	9
1	7	8	9	2	4	6	3	5
2	9	6	5	3	7	4	1	8

Puzzle 21 (Very hard, difficulty rating 0.84)

1	7	9	8	4	3	6	2	5
2	5	4	6	1	9	3	8	7
3	8	6	2	7	5	4	1	9
4	6	3	9	2	8	7	5	1
8	2	1	5	3	7	9	6	4
5	9	7	4	6	1	8	3	2
9	4	5	1	8	6	2	7	3
7	1	8	3	9	2	5	4	6
6	3	2	7	5	4	1	9	8

Puzzle 22 (Very hard, difficulty rating 0.87)

7	4	1	8	9	5	6	2	3
6	8	2	3	4	7	1	5	9
9	3	5	1	2	6	7	8	4
5	1	9	7	3	2	4	6	8
3	6	4	9	5	8	2	7	1
2	7	8	4	6	1	9	3	5
1	5	3	6	7	4	8	9	2
4	2	6	5	8	9	3	1	7
8	9	7	2	1	3	5	4	6

Puzzle 23 (Very hard, difficulty rating 0.90)

2	7	9	4	6	1	3	5	8
4	3	6	8	5	7	2	9	1
1	8	5	9	2	3	4	6	7
3	1	2	5	9	4	8	7	6
8	9	4	6	7	2	5	1	3
5	6	7	3	1	8	9	4	2
6	4	3	1	8	9	7	2	5
7	5	8	2	4	6	1	3	9
9	2	1	7	3	5	6	8	4

Puzzle 24 (Very hard, difficulty rating 0.79)

6	3	1	8	2	4	5	9	7
9	7	4	1	6	5	2	8	3
2	5	8	9	7	3	4	1	6
1	8	7	4	3	2	6	5	9
5	2	3	6	1	9	8	7	4
4	9	6	7	5	8	3	2	1
3	4	9	2	8	7	1	6	5
8	6	5	3	9	1	7	4	2
7	1	2	5	4	6	9	3	8

Puzzle 25 (Very hard, difficulty rating 0.82)

9	6	2	7	4	5	1	3	8
5	4	1	3	8	9	2	7	6
7	3	8	2	6	1	5	4	9
1	2	6	8	7	4	9	5	3
4	9	7	6	5	3	8	1	2
3	8	5	9	1	2	7	6	4
8	5	3	1	9	6	4	2	7
2	7	4	5	3	8	6	9	1
6	1	9	4	2	7	3	8	5

Puzzle 26 (Very hard, difficulty rating 0.82)

8	5	4	9	2	1	7	6	3
7	9	2	6	3	8	5	1	4
1	6	3	4	7	5	9	8	2
5	8	6	3	4	7	1	2	9
4	1	9	2	8	6	3	7	5
3	2	7	1	5	9	8	4	6
2	4	1	8	9	3	6	5	7
6	3	5	7	1	2	4	9	8
9	7	8	5	6	4	2	3	1

Puzzle 27 (Very hard, difficulty rating 0.93)

9	8	5	3	6	4	1	7	2
7	2	3	1	8	5	9	4	6
6	1	4	2	9	7	5	3	8
8	5	6	7	3	9	4	2	1
2	3	9	4	1	8	7	6	5
1	4	7	5	2	6	3	8	9
5	9	8	6	4	3	2	1	7
4	6	1	9	7	2	8	5	3
3	7	2	8	5	1	6	9	4

Puzzle 28 (Very hard, difficulty rating 0.86)

2	8	6	9	7	3	5	1	4
1	9	3	4	5	6	2	7	8
5	4	7	8	2	1	3	6	9
9	7	2	3	1	4	6	8	5
4	5	1	6	8	7	9	3	2
6	3	8	5	9	2	1	4	7
3	6	9	7	4	5	8	2	1
7	1	5	2	3	8	4	9	6
8	2	4	1	6	9	7	5	3

Puzzle 29 (Very hard, difficulty rating 0.79)

7	1	4	6	2	5	3	8	9
9	8	2	4	3	7	6	1	5
5	6	3	9	1	8	2	7	4
4	3	6	2	7	9	1	5	8
1	5	7	8	6	4	9	3	2
8	2	9	3	5	1	4	6	7
6	9	5	7	4	3	8	2	1
3	4	1	5	8	2	7	9	6
2	7	8	1	9	6	5	4	3

Puzzle 30 (Very hard, difficulty rating 0.83)

2	4	1	8	6	7	5	3	9
9	3	6	2	1	5	4	8	7
7	5	8	9	3	4	2	1	6
1	7	4	6	9	8	3	5	2
5	2	9	3	7	1	8	6	4
8	6	3	4	5	2	9	7	1
6	1	2	5	4	3	7	9	8
4	9	5	7	8	6	1	2	3
3	8	7	1	2	9	6	4	5

Puzzle 31 (Very hard, difficulty rating 0.80)

7	1	3	6	9	5	4	2	8
8	2	5	4	1	3	9	6	7
6	4	9	7	8	2	1	5	3
5	9	2	1	3	7	8	4	6
4	6	1	8	5	9	3	7	2
3	7	8	2	4	6	5	9	1
1	3	7	9	6	4	2	8	5
9	5	6	3	2	8	7	1	4
2	8	4	5	7	1	6	3	9

Puzzle 32 (Very hard, difficulty rating 0.90)

5	8	1	2	9	7	6	3	4
3	4	7	6	5	8	1	2	9
9	6	2	1	3	4	8	7	5
2	5	4	8	1	9	7	6	3
7	3	6	5	4	2	9	1	8
8	1	9	3	7	6	5	4	2
6	7	8	4	2	5	3	9	1
4	9	3	7	8	1	2	5	6
1	2	5	9	6	3	4	8	7

Puzzle 33 (Very hard, difficulty rating 0.87)

2	5	9	7	8	6	1	4	3
1	3	6	4	2	5	8	9	7
4	8	7	3	9	1	5	6	2
5	1	4	2	7	9	6	3	8
8	6	2	5	3	4	9	7	1
7	9	3	6	1	8	4	2	5
3	4	1	9	5	2	7	8	6
6	7	8	1	4	3	2	5	9
9	2	5	8	6	7	3	1	4

Puzzle 34 (Very hard, difficulty rating 0.79)

4	1	6	9	8	3	2	7	5
9	5	8	2	7	1	6	3	4
3	2	7	5	6	4	9	1	8
5	7	4	6	3	2	1	8	9
6	3	9	8	1	5	7	4	2
2	8	1	7	4	9	3	5	6
8	9	2	3	5	7	4	6	1
1	6	3	4	2	8	5	9	7
7	4	5	1	9	6	8	2	3

Puzzle 35 (Very hard, difficulty rating 0.84)

4	6	1	7	5	9	2	3	8
5	7	3	8	2	4	1	6	9
9	2	8	3	1	6	4	7	5
1	4	6	9	3	8	7	5	2
8	9	7	5	6	2	3	4	1
3	5	2	1	4	7	8	9	6
6	8	4	2	7	5	9	1	3
7	3	9	6	8	1	5	2	4
2	1	5	4	9	3	6	8	7

Puzzle 36 (Very hard, difficulty rating 0.83)

1	7	9	5	3	6	4	8	2
3	5	8	2	4	7	9	6	1
6	4	2	8	1	9	5	3	7
5	1	7	3	9	2	6	4	8
4	8	6	7	5	1	3	2	9
9	2	3	4	6	8	7	1	5
7	3	4	1	8	5	2	9	6
8	9	5	6	2	3	1	7	4
2	6	1	9	7	4	8	5	3

Puzzle 37 (Very hard, difficulty rating 0.75)

5	1	9	2	4	6	7	3	8
6	7	4	3	5	8	9	2	1
2	3	8	9	7	1	5	4	6
8	9	1	4	3	5	2	6	7
3	2	6	1	9	7	4	8	5
4	5	7	8	6	2	3	1	9
1	8	3	7	2	9	6	5	4
9	4	5	6	1	3	8	7	2
7	6	2	5	8	4	1	9	3

Puzzle 38 (Very hard, difficulty rating 0.76)

9	2	8	6	3	4	1	5	7
7	5	3	9	2	1	8	6	4
4	1	6	5	7	8	9	2	3
3	4	5	7	6	9	2	1	8
1	8	7	2	4	5	6	3	9
2	6	9	8	1	3	4	7	5
5	9	2	3	8	6	7	4	1
6	3	4	1	9	7	5	8	2
8	7	1	4	5	2	3	9	6

Puzzle 39 (Very hard, difficulty rating 0.79)

1	4	7	2	6	5	9	3	8
2	9	5	8	1	3	6	4	7
6	8	3	7	9	4	1	5	2
3	5	1	9	8	6	7	2	4
7	2	9	3	4	1	8	6	5
4	6	8	5	7	2	3	9	1
9	3	4	1	2	7	5	8	6
8	1	2	6	5	9	4	7	3
5	7	6	4	3	8	2	1	9

Puzzle 40 (Very hard, difficulty rating 0.80)

5	8	2	9	7	3	6	1	4
7	9	3	6	4	1	5	8	2
6	4	1	2	8	5	3	9	7
9	5	8	7	2	4	1	6	3
1	2	4	3	9	6	7	5	8
3	7	6	5	1	8	4	2	9
8	6	9	1	3	7	2	4	5
4	3	5	8	6	2	9	7	1
2	1	7	4	5	9	8	3	6

Puzzle 41 (Very hard, difficulty rating 0.84)

7	6	4	5	3	1	8	2	9
1	2	3	7	8	9	5	6	4
9	5	8	4	2	6	7	3	1
4	9	6	1	7	2	3	5	8
5	1	2	8	6	3	9	4	7
3	8	7	9	5	4	6	1	2
2	3	9	6	1	8	4	7	5
6	4	5	2	9	7	1	8	3
8	7	1	3	4	5	2	9	6

Puzzle 42 (Very hard, difficulty rating 0.88)

9	2	4	8	7	5	1	3	6
5	1	8	2	3	6	9	7	4
7	6	3	4	1	9	5	2	8
6	9	2	5	8	3	7	4	1
4	5	1	7	6	2	8	9	3
3	8	7	9	4	1	2	6	5
8	7	6	1	9	4	3	5	2
2	3	9	6	5	8	4	1	7
1	4	5	3	2	7	6	8	9

Puzzle 43 (Very hard, difficulty rating 0.81)

8	5	1	7	2	9	6	4	3
3	9	7	5	6	4	2	8	1
4	2	6	8	3	1	5	7	9
5	6	9	2	4	7	3	1	8
1	3	2	9	5	8	7	6	4
7	4	8	6	1	3	9	5	2
9	8	5	4	7	2	1	3	6
2	7	3	1	8	6	4	9	5
6	1	4	3	9	5	8	2	7

Puzzle 44 (Very hard, difficulty rating 0.80)

5	9	8	6	1	2	3	4	7
2	1	7	9	3	4	8	6	5
6	4	3	5	8	7	1	2	9
1	6	5	4	9	8	2	7	3
3	2	9	7	6	5	4	1	8
7	8	4	3	2	1	5	9	6
8	3	1	2	7	6	9	5	4
4	7	2	8	5	9	6	3	1
9	5	6	1	4	3	7	8	2

Puzzle 45 (Very hard, difficulty rating 0.80)

4	3	8	1	7	6	9	2	5
7	9	2	5	8	4	6	3	1
5	6	1	9	2	3	8	7	4
6	1	3	7	4	5	2	9	8
2	5	4	8	3	9	7	1	6
9	8	7	6	1	2	5	4	3
3	7	5	4	9	8	1	6	2
1	2	6	3	5	7	4	8	9
8	4	9	2	6	1	3	5	7

Puzzle 46 (Very hard, difficulty rating 0.78)

1	3	7	9	8	4	2	6	5
6	4	9	2	1	5	3	7	8
2	5	8	6	7	3	9	1	4
7	1	5	8	9	2	4	3	6
8	2	4	7	3	6	1	5	9
9	6	3	4	5	1	7	8	2
3	7	6	5	2	9	8	4	1
5	9	1	3	4	8	6	2	7
4	8	2	1	6	7	5	9	3

Puzzle 47 (Very hard, difficulty rating 0.80)

8	6	9	4	7	3	1	2	5
4	3	7	2	5	1	9	8	6
5	2	1	9	8	6	4	3	7
7	1	8	6	9	5	2	4	3
6	4	3	7	1	2	8	5	9
9	5	2	3	4	8	6	7	1
1	9	5	8	2	7	3	6	4
2	7	6	1	3	4	5	9	8
3	8	4	5	6	9	7	1	2

Puzzle 48 (Very hard, difficulty rating 0.81)

3	1	4	5	9	8	2	7	6
6	2	8	1	7	3	9	4	5
9	7	5	4	6	2	8	1	3
7	8	6	3	4	5	1	9	2
1	3	9	2	8	7	5	6	4
4	5	2	9	1	6	3	8	7
2	6	7	8	5	1	4	3	9
5	4	1	6	3	9	7	2	8
8	9	3	7	2	4	6	5	1

Puzzle 49 (Very hard, difficulty rating 0.80)

1	6	2	4	7	9	3	5	8
9	7	3	8	5	1	6	2	4
4	5	8	2	6	3	9	7	1
3	2	5	1	8	6	4	9	7
6	9	4	5	3	7	1	8	2
7	8	1	9	4	2	5	6	3
5	1	7	6	2	4	8	3	9
2	4	6	3	9	8	7	1	5
8	3	9	7	1	5	2	4	6

Puzzle 50 (Very hard, difficulty rating 0.79)

9	4	5	3	7	1	2	6	8
3	7	1	8	6	2	5	9	4
2	6	8	5	9	4	7	3	1
4	9	6	2	8	5	3	1	7
1	5	3	6	4	7	9	8	2
7	8	2	1	3	9	4	5	6
5	2	9	4	1	6	8	7	3
6	3	7	9	2	8	1	4	5
8	1	4	7	5	3	6	2	9

DIFFICULTY LEVEL: RANDOM

Puzzle 1 (Hard, difficulty rating 0.73)

9	7	8	2	6	1	3	5	4
5	4	6	7	3	8	2	9	1
1	2	3	9	5	4	8	7	6
7	8	4	1	2	3	5	6	9
6	3	1	5	4	9	7	2	8
2	5	9	6	8	7	1	4	3
8	9	5	3	7	6	4	1	2
4	1	2	8	9	5	6	3	7
3	6	7	4	1	2	9	8	5

Puzzle 2 (Easy, difficulty rating 0.36)

5	2	3	4	1	6	8	9	7
9	7	6	3	2	8	4	5	1
1	8	4	7	5	9	6	3	2
4	3	2	1	8	7	5	6	9
7	5	9	6	4	2	3	1	8
8	6	1	9	3	5	2	7	4
6	1	5	2	9	4	7	8	3
2	9	8	5	7	3	1	4	6
3	4	7	8	6	1	9	2	5

Puzzle 3 (Hard, difficulty rating 0.67)

6	9	8	4	5	3	2	7	1
5	4	3	2	1	7	9	6	8
2	7	1	9	8	6	3	5	4
9	5	2	1	6	8	7	4	3
4	1	7	3	2	9	5	8	6
3	8	6	5	7	4	1	2	9
7	2	4	6	9	1	8	3	5
1	3	5	8	4	2	6	9	7
8	6	9	7	3	5	4	1	2

Puzzle 4 (Easy, difficulty rating 0.37)

1	6	8	9	7	3	2	5	4
9	5	7	2	4	1	6	8	3
2	3	4	6	5	8	1	9	7
8	2	5	4	1	6	3	7	9
3	1	6	7	9	5	4	2	8
4	7	9	3	8	2	5	6	1
7	9	1	5	2	4	8	3	6
5	8	3	1	6	9	7	4	2
6	4	2	8	3	7	9	1	5

Puzzle 5 (Medium, difficulty rating 0.52)

7	6	5	3	1	2	4	8	9
2	4	8	9	6	5	7	1	3
3	1	9	7	4	8	6	2	5
4	2	3	5	7	9	8	6	1
5	8	1	4	2	6	3	9	7
9	7	6	8	3	1	5	4	2
6	3	7	2	9	4	1	5	8
8	9	4	1	5	3	2	7	6
1	5	2	6	8	7	9	3	4

Puzzle 6 (Easy, difficulty rating 0.21)

3	5	8	7	9	4	2	6	1
1	7	6	2	8	5	9	4	3
4	2	9	6	3	1	8	7	5
7	3	2	8	1	6	5	9	4
9	1	5	3	4	7	6	8	2
8	6	4	5	2	9	3	1	7
5	9	7	1	6	3	4	2	8
6	8	3	4	7	2	1	5	9
2	4	1	9	5	8	7	3	6

Puzzle 7 (Hard, difficulty rating 0.61)

3	4	9	5	8	6	2	7	1
2	5	7	1	3	4	9	6	8
8	1	6	9	2	7	4	3	5
1	6	5	7	4	9	8	2	3
9	7	3	2	6	8	5	1	4
4	2	8	3	1	5	7	9	6
5	3	2	8	7	1	6	4	9
7	9	4	6	5	3	1	8	2
6	8	1	4	9	2	3	5	7

Puzzle 8 (Medium, difficulty rating 0.49)

6	8	5	7	4	2	1	9	3
1	7	9	3	5	6	8	4	2
2	3	4	9	8	1	6	7	5
7	6	1	5	2	9	3	8	4
9	2	8	4	1	3	5	6	7
4	5	3	8	6	7	2	1	9
3	1	6	2	9	4	7	5	8
8	9	2	1	7	5	4	3	6
5	4	7	6	3	8	9	2	1

Puzzle 9 (Very hard, difficulty rating 0.77)

1	3	4	5	2	6	7	9	8
7	2	5	4	8	9	6	1	3
6	9	8	3	7	1	4	2	5
4	7	3	2	5	8	1	6	9
5	1	9	6	3	4	8	7	2
8	6	2	9	1	7	5	3	4
3	8	7	1	9	5	2	4	6
9	4	1	8	6	2	3	5	7
2	5	6	7	4	3	9	8	1

Puzzle 10 (Medium, difficulty rating 0.48)

4	9	3	6	5	7	1	8	2
5	1	8	2	4	9	6	7	3
6	2	7	1	3	8	5	9	4
9	8	6	5	7	4	3	2	1
3	5	1	8	2	6	7	4	9
7	4	2	9	1	3	8	6	5
8	3	5	7	9	2	4	1	6
2	7	4	3	6	1	9	5	8
1	6	9	4	8	5	2	3	7

Puzzle 11 (Easy, difficulty rating 0.43)

5	9	6	7	8	1	4	3	2
4	2	8	6	3	9	1	7	5
1	7	3	2	5	4	8	9	6
3	5	4	9	6	8	2	1	7
9	8	1	5	7	2	6	4	3
2	6	7	1	4	3	9	5	8
6	3	9	8	1	5	7	2	4
8	4	2	3	9	7	5	6	1
7	1	5	4	2	6	3	8	9

Puzzle 12 (Easy, difficulty rating 0.34)

2	1	8	5	4	9	3	7	6
4	3	5	6	1	7	9	8	2
9	6	7	8	3	2	5	1	4
6	5	9	7	8	4	1	2	3
7	4	1	2	9	3	8	6	5
8	2	3	1	5	6	4	9	7
1	8	2	3	6	5	7	4	9
3	7	4	9	2	1	6	5	8
5	9	6	4	7	8	2	3	1

Puzzle 13 (Easy, difficulty rating 0.37)

8	5	7	1	2	3	6	9	4
6	1	4	9	5	7	8	3	2
9	3	2	4	6	8	1	5	7
4	8	9	7	3	1	2	6	5
1	2	3	5	8	6	4	7	9
5	7	6	2	4	9	3	1	8
3	6	5	8	7	2	9	4	1
2	4	1	6	9	5	7	8	3
7	9	8	3	1	4	5	2	6

Puzzle 14 (Hard, difficulty rating 0.61)

5	3	6	8	1	7	9	4	2
9	8	4	6	5	2	3	1	7
7	2	1	3	9	4	6	5	8
8	9	5	4	3	6	7	2	1
6	4	7	5	2	1	8	3	9
2	1	3	7	8	9	4	6	5
4	6	8	1	7	5	2	9	3
1	7	2	9	4	3	5	8	6
3	5	9	2	6	8	1	7	4

Puzzle 15 (Very hard, difficulty rating 0.83)

6	4	3	1	2	7	5	8	9
9	5	7	8	4	6	2	3	1
2	1	8	3	5	9	6	7	4
3	8	4	7	1	2	9	6	5
5	6	1	9	3	4	7	2	8
7	9	2	5	6	8	4	1	3
4	7	5	6	8	1	3	9	2
1	2	9	4	7	3	8	5	6
8	3	6	2	9	5	1	4	7

Puzzle 16 (Hard, difficulty rating 0.69)

7	4	9	6	2	8	5	3	1
5	6	2	7	3	1	9	4	8
3	1	8	5	4	9	7	6	2
8	2	1	3	9	5	6	7	4
4	3	6	1	7	2	8	5	9
9	7	5	4	8	6	1	2	3
6	9	7	2	1	3	4	8	5
2	8	4	9	5	7	3	1	6
1	5	3	8	6	4	2	9	7

Puzzle 17 (Medium, difficulty rating 0.52)

1	6	4	7	5	9	2	3	8
2	8	9	3	6	1	5	7	4
3	7	5	8	2	4	9	1	6
5	4	1	2	9	3	6	8	7
9	3	6	1	8	7	4	5	2
7	2	8	5	4	6	1	9	3
6	9	7	4	3	5	8	2	1
8	5	3	6	1	2	7	4	9
4	1	2	9	7	8	3	6	5

Puzzle 18 (Hard, difficulty rating 0.67)

5	9	6	7	8	1	4	3	2
4	2	8	6	3	9	1	7	5
1	7	3	2	5	4	8	9	6
3	5	4	9	6	8	2	1	7
9	8	1	5	7	2	6	4	3
2	6	7	1	4	3	9	5	8
6	3	9	8	1	5	7	2	4
8	4	2	3	9	7	5	6	1
7	1	5	4	2	6	3	8	9

Puzzle 19 (Very hard, difficulty rating 0.89)

2	1	8	4	5	9	3	6	7
4	7	3	8	6	1	5	9	2
9	5	6	7	2	3	8	1	4
3	4	2	5	1	6	7	8	9
7	6	9	2	3	8	1	4	5
5	8	1	9	4	7	6	2	3
8	3	5	6	9	2	4	7	1
1	2	7	3	8	4	9	5	6
6	9	4	1	7	5	2	3	8

Puzzle 20 (Medium, difficulty rating 0.56)

4	2	6	1	3	5	7	8	9
3	8	9	6	4	7	1	5	2
5	7	1	9	8	2	4	6	3
2	4	8	7	9	6	5	3	1
6	1	5	8	2	3	9	7	4
7	9	3	5	1	4	6	2	8
9	6	4	3	5	8	2	1	7
8	5	2	4	7	1	3	9	6
1	3	7	2	6	9	8	4	5

Puzzle 21 (Easy, difficulty rating 0.43)

5	4	1	9	7	3	8	2	6
9	3	2	5	6	8	4	7	1
8	6	7	1	2	4	9	3	5
7	8	9	4	3	5	1	6	2
6	2	3	8	1	7	5	4	9
1	5	4	6	9	2	3	8	7
3	7	8	2	5	1	6	9	4
4	1	6	7	8	9	2	5	3
2	9	5	3	4	6	7	1	8

Puzzle 22 (Easy, difficulty rating 0.44)

8	2	4	1	6	3	9	7	5
6	7	1	9	4	5	8	2	3
5	3	9	7	2	8	6	1	4
1	5	3	6	8	9	2	4	7
2	6	8	4	7	1	5	3	9
4	9	7	3	5	2	1	8	6
9	4	2	5	1	7	3	6	8
3	1	6	8	9	4	7	5	2
7	8	5	2	3	6	4	9	1

Puzzle 23 (Medium, difficulty rating 0.47)

2	3	4	8	6	7	1	5	9
5	6	9	3	1	4	8	7	2
7	8	1	2	9	5	3	6	4
8	2	7	5	4	1	6	9	3
4	1	5	9	3	6	7	2	8
3	9	6	7	2	8	5	4	1
6	5	3	4	8	2	9	1	7
9	7	2	1	5	3	4	8	6
1	4	8	6	7	9	2	3	5

Puzzle 24 (Easy, difficulty rating 0.43)

1	8	2	7	6	9	3	4	5
9	6	7	3	5	4	2	1	8
5	4	3	1	2	8	7	9	6
4	1	8	2	7	6	5	3	9
7	9	5	4	8	3	6	2	1
2	3	6	9	1	5	4	8	7
6	2	4	5	9	1	8	7	3
8	7	9	6	3	2	1	5	4
3	5	1	8	4	7	9	6	2

Puzzle 25 (Easy, difficulty rating 0.41)

3	4	5	1	8	2	7	6	9
7	9	8	5	6	4	3	1	2
6	1	2	9	3	7	8	4	5
8	3	1	4	9	5	2	7	6
4	7	6	8	2	3	5	9	1
2	5	9	6	7	1	4	3	8
5	2	3	7	1	9	6	8	4
9	8	4	3	5	6	1	2	7
1	6	7	2	4	8	9	5	3

Puzzle 26 (Medium, difficulty rating 0.48)

4	6	7	1	2	5	8	3	9
2	8	3	4	9	7	1	6	5
5	1	9	8	6	3	2	7	4
6	5	8	9	7	2	3	4	1
9	7	4	3	1	6	5	8	2
3	2	1	5	8	4	7	9	6
7	3	5	6	4	1	9	2	8
8	4	2	7	5	9	6	1	3
1	9	6	2	3	8	4	5	7

Puzzle 27 (Easy, difficulty rating 0.42)

1	9	3	5	7	2	4	8	6
6	2	4	3	8	9	5	1	7
8	5	7	4	1	6	9	3	2
9	8	2	1	6	7	3	5	4
7	4	1	9	3	5	2	6	8
3	6	5	2	4	8	1	7	9
5	3	8	7	2	4	6	9	1
4	1	6	8	9	3	7	2	5
2	7	9	6	5	1	8	4	3

Puzzle 28 (Very hard, difficulty rating 0.79)

3	8	5	4	1	9	6	7	2
7	6	1	3	8	2	9	5	4
9	2	4	5	6	7	8	1	3
8	5	9	2	4	1	3	6	7
4	1	7	9	3	6	2	8	5
6	3	2	7	5	8	1	4	9
1	7	3	8	2	5	4	9	6
5	4	8	6	9	3	7	2	1
2	9	6	1	7	4	5	3	8

Puzzle 29 (Hard, difficulty rating 0.60)

8	2	5	7	6	1	9	3	4
1	3	4	2	5	9	7	8	6
9	7	6	8	3	4	2	1	5
4	5	9	1	8	6	3	2	7
6	1	3	4	2	7	8	5	9
2	8	7	3	9	5	4	6	1
3	9	1	5	4	2	6	7	8
5	6	2	9	7	8	1	4	3
7	4	8	6	1	3	5	9	2

Puzzle 30 (Medium, difficulty rating 0.57)

5	3	2	8	4	1	7	9	6
4	6	7	5	2	9	3	8	1
1	9	8	3	7	6	5	2	4
8	2	6	7	5	3	1	4	9
3	4	9	1	6	2	8	7	5
7	5	1	9	8	4	6	3	2
2	8	4	6	1	7	9	5	3
9	1	5	4	3	8	2	6	7
6	7	3	2	9	5	4	1	8

Puzzle 31 (Medium, difficulty rating 0.52)

8	4	1	3	5	6	2	7	9
6	5	2	7	9	4	8	3	1
3	9	7	8	2	1	5	4	6
7	6	5	2	3	8	9	1	4
2	1	4	6	7	9	3	8	5
9	8	3	4	1	5	7	6	2
5	3	6	1	8	2	4	9	7
4	7	9	5	6	3	1	2	8
1	2	8	9	4	7	6	5	3

Puzzle 32 (Very hard, difficulty rating 0.77)

2	6	5	4	7	3	8	9	1
9	3	8	2	6	1	7	5	4
4	1	7	5	9	8	3	6	2
1	9	6	7	2	5	4	3	8
3	7	2	6	8	4	5	1	9
8	5	4	3	1	9	2	7	6
5	2	1	8	3	6	9	4	7
7	4	9	1	5	2	6	8	3
6	8	3	9	4	7	1	2	5

Puzzle 33 (Medium, difficulty rating 0.49)

8	6	1	4	2	7	3	9	5
5	4	2	8	9	3	1	6	7
9	7	3	1	6	5	4	2	8
2	1	9	7	8	4	6	5	3
7	3	8	9	5	6	2	4	1
6	5	4	2	3	1	8	7	9
4	8	6	3	7	9	5	1	2
3	9	5	6	1	2	7	8	4
1	2	7	5	4	8	9	3	6

Puzzle 34 (Medium, difficulty rating 0.51)

2	8	9	5	1	4	3	6	7
6	3	4	7	8	2	9	5	1
5	1	7	6	3	9	4	8	2
7	9	5	4	6	8	2	1	3
1	2	6	3	9	7	8	4	5
3	4	8	1	2	5	7	9	6
8	6	1	2	4	3	5	7	9
9	7	2	8	5	6	1	3	4
4	5	3	9	7	1	6	2	8

Puzzle 35 (Medium, difficulty rating 0.57)

5	3	2	7	4	1	6	9	8
9	4	6	8	2	3	7	5	1
8	7	1	5	9	6	4	2	3
2	9	3	4	6	8	1	7	5
1	6	7	2	3	5	8	4	9
4	8	5	1	7	9	3	6	2
3	5	9	6	8	7	2	1	4
6	1	4	3	5	2	9	8	7
7	2	8	9	1	4	5	3	6

Puzzle 36 (Easy, difficulty rating 0.36)

4	2	6	9	7	3	1	8	5
7	9	8	6	5	1	2	4	3
3	5	1	2	4	8	9	6	7
8	3	9	7	2	4	6	5	1
6	1	2	8	3	5	4	7	9
5	7	4	1	6	9	8	3	2
1	4	7	3	8	2	5	9	6
2	6	5	4	9	7	3	1	8
9	8	3	5	1	6	7	2	4

Puzzle 37 (Easy, difficulty rating 0.41)

5	3	8	6	7	9	1	4	2
4	7	9	2	8	1	5	6	3
6	2	1	5	4	3	9	7	8
9	1	6	8	2	7	4	3	5
8	5	2	4	3	6	7	9	1
7	4	3	9	1	5	8	2	6
1	8	7	3	9	2	6	5	4
3	6	4	7	5	8	2	1	9
2	9	5	1	6	4	3	8	7

Puzzle 38 (Easy, difficulty rating 0.43)

6	1	5	3	8	2	7	4	9
3	8	4	9	5	7	1	2	6
9	7	2	4	6	1	8	5	3
4	5	6	2	1	3	9	8	7
7	9	1	8	4	5	3	6	2
8	2	3	7	9	6	4	1	5
2	4	8	6	7	9	5	3	1
5	3	7	1	2	4	6	9	8
1	6	9	5	3	8	2	7	4

Puzzle 39 (Medium, difficulty rating 0.51)

6	8	5	3	7	2	1	4	9
7	2	1	9	8	4	5	3	6
4	9	3	6	1	5	2	7	8
9	3	4	1	5	6	7	8	2
1	7	8	2	4	9	6	5	3
5	6	2	8	3	7	4	9	1
2	5	6	7	9	3	8	1	4
8	4	9	5	2	1	3	6	7
3	1	7	4	6	8	9	2	5

Puzzle 40 (Easy, difficulty rating 0.44)

5	6	4	2	9	3	1	7	8
7	8	2	1	5	4	6	3	9
9	3	1	8	7	6	2	5	4
8	7	5	4	6	1	3	9	2
4	2	9	3	8	7	5	6	1
6	1	3	9	2	5	4	8	7
3	9	8	5	1	2	7	4	6
2	5	6	7	4	8	9	1	3
1	4	7	6	3	9	8	2	5

Puzzle 41 (Medium, difficulty rating 0.49)

1	6	7	5	2	4	9	3	8
2	3	9	1	7	8	6	5	4
8	5	4	3	9	6	2	7	1
6	9	8	7	4	2	3	1	5
7	2	3	6	1	5	4	8	9
5	4	1	8	3	9	7	6	2
3	1	2	4	8	7	5	9	6
9	7	6	2	5	1	8	4	3
4	8	5	9	6	3	1	2	7

Puzzle 42 (Easy, difficulty rating 0.41)

7	4	1	2	6	5	8	9	3
8	6	9	3	1	7	4	2	5
5	2	3	4	9	8	1	7	6
9	5	6	7	8	2	3	1	4
2	7	4	1	5	3	9	6	8
3	1	8	6	4	9	7	5	2
6	9	2	8	3	1	5	4	7
1	8	7	5	2	4	6	3	9
4	3	5	9	7	6	2	8	1

Puzzle 43 (Medium, difficulty rating 0.55)

4	5	2	3	9	6	1	7	8
1	9	3	5	7	8	4	6	2
7	8	6	2	4	1	5	9	3
2	6	9	4	3	7	8	1	5
3	7	4	8	1	5	9	2	6
5	1	8	6	2	9	3	4	7
6	2	1	9	8	3	7	5	4
9	3	5	7	6	4	2	8	1
8	4	7	1	5	2	6	3	9

Puzzle 44 (Easy, difficulty rating 0.31)

1	7	9	8	4	3	6	2	5
2	5	4	6	1	9	3	8	7
3	8	6	2	7	5	4	1	9
4	6	3	9	2	8	7	5	1
8	2	1	5	3	7	9	6	4
5	9	7	4	6	1	8	3	2
9	4	5	1	8	6	2	7	3
7	1	8	3	9	2	5	4	6
6	3	2	7	5	4	1	9	8

Puzzle 45 (Medium, difficulty rating 0.50)

7	4	9	1	2	5	3	8	6
2	5	1	6	8	3	9	4	7
3	8	6	4	9	7	1	5	2
8	1	7	2	5	6	4	3	9
5	2	4	7	3	9	8	6	1
9	6	3	8	1	4	2	7	5
4	3	2	5	6	1	7	9	8
6	9	8	3	7	2	5	1	4
1	7	5	9	4	8	6	2	3

Puzzle 46 (Easy, difficulty rating 0.41)

1	3	7	8	6	9	4	2	5
5	8	6	1	4	2	3	9	7
4	9	2	3	7	5	1	8	6
6	7	3	5	8	1	2	4	9
2	5	8	4	9	3	6	7	1
9	1	4	6	2	7	5	3	8
8	6	9	2	1	4	7	5	3
3	4	1	7	5	8	9	6	2
7	2	5	9	3	6	8	1	4

Puzzle 47 (Hard, difficulty rating 0.70)

1	9	3	4	6	7	8	5	2
5	7	2	9	3	8	1	4	6
4	8	6	1	5	2	7	3	9
6	1	7	3	9	4	5	2	8
9	4	8	2	7	5	3	6	1
3	2	5	8	1	6	9	7	4
7	3	1	6	2	9	4	8	5
8	6	9	5	4	3	2	1	7
2	5	4	7	8	1	6	9	3

Puzzle 48 (Medium, difficulty rating 0.59)

7	4	6	1	5	9	8	3	2
8	5	3	6	2	4	9	1	7
1	2	9	3	7	8	6	4	5
6	7	8	5	9	3	1	2	4
4	3	2	7	1	6	5	8	9
9	1	5	4	8	2	7	6	3
5	6	7	2	3	1	4	9	8
2	8	4	9	6	5	3	7	1
3	9	1	8	4	7	2	5	6

Puzzle 49 (Medium, difficulty rating 0.59)

1	8	5	7	9	6	2	4	3
7	2	9	8	4	3	6	1	5
6	4	3	1	2	5	7	8	9
2	3	4	5	6	7	1	9	8
5	9	7	4	1	8	3	2	6
8	1	6	2	3	9	4	5	7
9	5	1	6	7	4	8	3	2
3	6	2	9	8	1	5	7	4
4	7	8	3	5	2	9	6	1

Puzzle 50 (Medium, difficulty rating 0.52)

7	6	2	3	1	9	4	8	5
9	4	3	5	8	6	7	1	2
5	8	1	7	2	4	6	9	3
6	3	4	9	7	5	1	2	8
1	9	7	8	3	2	5	6	4
2	5	8	4	6	1	3	7	9
3	2	5	1	9	7	8	4	6
8	1	9	6	4	3	2	5	7
4	7	6	2	5	8	9	3	1

RELATED SUDOKU BOOKS

	Easy-to-Hard Sudoku Vol. 1: 250 Puzzles of Mixed Difficulty Levels Dimensions: 8" x 10" ISBN-13: 978-1533168184
	Easy-to-Hard Sudoku Vol. 2: 250 Puzzles of Mixed Difficulty Levels Dimensions: 8" x 10" Scheduled for Release: June 2016
	Travel Sudoku Vol. 1: 200 Easy to Hard Puzzles Dimensions: 5.25" x 8" ISBN-13: 978-1533400659
	Travel Sudoku Vol. 2: 200 Easy to Hard Puzzles Dimensions: 5.25" x 8" Scheduled for Release: June 2016

Note: Puzzles are all unique in the various editions and volumes.

www.ingramcontent.com/pod-product-compliance
Lightning Source LLC
Chambersburg PA
CBHW080620190526
45169CB00009B/3250

* 9 7 8 1 5 3 3 1 6 8 1 8 4 *